MW01686700

SCIENTOLOGY

Improving Life in a Troubled World

Founded and developed by L. Ron Hubbard, Scientology is an applied religious philosophy which offers an exact route through which anyone can regain the truth and simplicity of his spiritual self.

Scientology consists of specific axioms that define the underlying causes and principles of existence and a vast area of observations in the humanities, a philosophic body that literally applies to the entirety of life.

This broad body of knowledge resulted in two applications of the subject: first, a technology for man to increase his spiritual awareness and attain the freedom sought by many great philosophic teachings; and, second, a great number of fundamental principles men can use to improve their lives. In fact, in this second application, Scientology offers nothing less than practical methods to better *every* aspect of our existence—means to create new ways of life. And from this comes the subject matter you are about to read.

Compiled from the writings of L. Ron Hubbard, the data presented here is but one of the tools which can be found in *The Scientology Handbook*. A comprehensive guide, the handbook contains numerous applications of Scientology which can be used to improve many other areas of life.

In this booklet, the editors have augmented the data with a short introduction, practical exercises and examples of successful application.

Courses to increase your understanding and further materials to broaden your knowledge are available at your nearest Scientology church or mission, listed at the back of this booklet.

Many new phenomena about man and life are described in Scientology, and so you may encounter terms in these pages you are not familiar with. These are described the first time they appear and in the glossary at the back of the booklet.

Scientology is for use. It is a practical philosophy, something one *does*. Using this data, you *can* change conditions.

Millions of people who want to do something about the conditions they see around them have applied this knowledge. They know that life can be improved. And they know that Scientology works.

Use what you read in these pages to help yourself and others and you will too.

CHURCH OF SCIENTOLOGY INTERNATIONAL

To say that drugs have become the major affliction of society is not stating the situation too strongly. No sector of life is untouched by this epidemic. Crime and violence are the most obvious byproducts, but amorality, aborted educations and, indeed, ruined lives are no less serious and just as widespread.

And the problem is not limited to street drugs; the effects of medical and psychiatric drugs, whether painkillers, tranquilizers or "antidepressants," are as disastrous.

L. Ron Hubbard addressed this problem, not with the objective of resolving the physical ills of individuals but as a continuation of his quest to free man as a spirit and handle, along this route, any barrier that needed to be resolved. Drugs were such a barrier.

Until Mr. Hubbard developed a workable drug rehabilitation program, there was no solution. Psychiatric-inspired programs had many more failures than successes and some only created worse addictions. Other people, more well-intentioned, found that good intentions weren't enough. They lacked a technology that worked.

Mr. Hubbard's program provides that technology. From helping the person discover why he took drugs in the first place, to eliminating the mental and spiritual damage done by drugs, to detoxifying the body of long-term drug residues, to providing the person with tools that will enable him to stay off drugs for good, it is without doubt the most thorough and effective program in the world. Today, for the first time, as hundreds of thousands will attest, those addicted to drugs and alcohol can free themselves of this tyranny and face life with renewed vigor and hope. This booklet contains some of the elementary principles of this program and provides the first real understanding of substance abuse problems.

The Reason Behind the Drug Problem

People have used drugs for as long as they have tried to ease pain and avoid problems. Since the early 1960s, however, drugs have been in very widespread use. Before that time they were rare. A worldwide spread of drugs occurred during that decade, and a large percentage of people became drug-takers.

By drugs (to mention a few) are meant tranquilizers, opium, cocaine, marijuana, peyote, amphetamines and the psychiatrist's gifts to man, LSD and angel dust, which are the worst. Any medical drugs are included. Drugs are drugs. There are thousands of trade names and slang terms for these drugs. Alcohol is also classified as a drug.

Drugs are supposed to do wonderful things but all they really do is ruin the person.

Drug problems do not end when a person stops taking drugs. The accumulated effects of drug-taking can leave one severely impaired, both physically and mentally. Even someone off drugs for years still has "blank periods." Drugs can injure a person's ability to concentrate, to work, to learn—in short, they can shatter a life.

Yet though the dangers and liabilities of drugs are blatantly obvious and increasingly well documented, people continue to take them.

Why?

When a person is depressed or in pain, and where he finds no physical relief from treatment, he will eventually discover for himself that drugs remove his symptoms.

This is also true for pains which are "psychosomatic." The term "psychosomatic" means the mind making the body ill or illnesses caused through the mind. "Psycho" refers to "mind" and "soma" refers to "body."

In almost all cases of psychosomatic pain, illness or discomfort the person has sought some cure for the upset.

When he at last finds that only drugs give him relief, he will surrender to them and become dependent upon them, often to the point of addiction.

Years before, had there been any other way out, most people would have taken it. But when they are told there is no cure, that their pains are "imaginary," life tends to become insupportable. They then can become chronic drug-takers and are in danger of addiction.

The time required to make an addict varies, of course. The complaint itself may only be "sadness" or "weariness." The ability to face life, in any case, is reduced.

Any substance that brings relief or makes life less a burden physically or mentally will then be welcome.

In an unsettled and insecure environment, psychosomatic illness is very widespread.

So before any government strikes too heavily at spreading drug use, it should recognize that it is a symptom of failed psychotherapy. The social scientist, the psychologist and psychiatrist and health ministers have failed to handle spreading psychosomatic illness.

It is too easy to blame the drug problem on "social unrest" or the "pace of modern society."

The hard, solid fact is that until now there has been no effective psychotherapy in broad practice. The result is a drug-dependent population.

Drug users have been found to have begun taking drugs because of physical suffering or hopelessness.

The user, driven by pain and environmental hopelessness, continues to take drugs. Though he doesn't want to be an addict, he doesn't feel that there is any other way out.

However, with proper treatment, drug dependency *can* be fully handled.

As soon as he can feel healthier and more competent mentally and physically without drugs than he does on drugs, a person ceases to require drugs.

Drug addiction has been shrugged off by psychiatry as "unimportant" and the social problem of drug-taking has received no attention from psychiatrists—rather the contrary, since they themselves introduced and popularized LSD. And many of them are pushers.

Government agencies have failed markedly to halt the increase in drug-taking and there has been no real or widespread cure.

The liability of the drug user, even after he has ceased to use drugs, is that he "goes blank" at unexpected times, has periods of irresponsibility and tends to sicken easily.

Scientology technology has been able to eradicate the major damage in persons who have been on drugs as well as make further addiction unnecessary and unwanted.

Scientology has no interest in the political or social aspects of the various types of drugs or even drug-taking as such. Drugs, however, pose a growing threat to mental and spiritual advancement—which is the true mission of Scientology.

Thus, Scientology contains an exact technology which not only gets a person painlessly off drugs but handles their physical, mental and spiritual effects *and* locates and fully resolves the reason underlying a person's drug-taking. Nothing else can do this with certainty.

When a person can find no solution to a problem, whether the problem be anything from physical suffering to hopelessness . . .

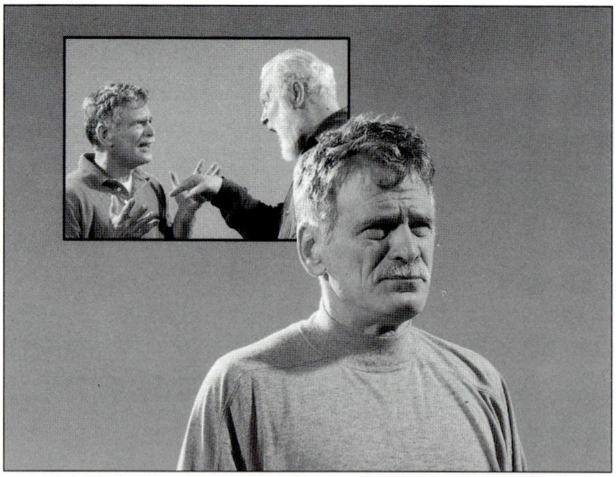

. . . he sooner or later finds that drugs relieve symptoms.

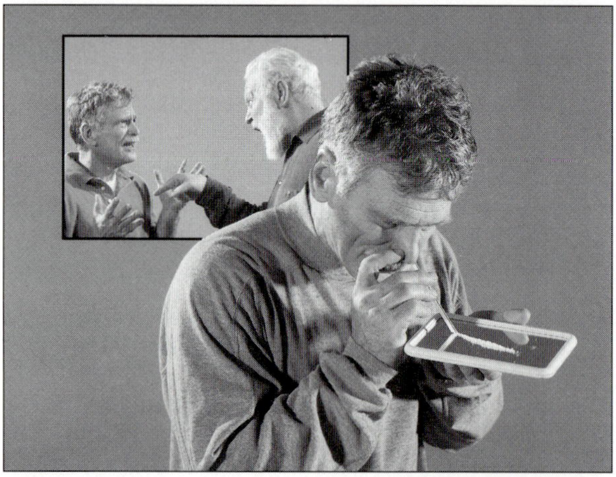

The problem, however, is not gone, but only masked by the drugs. Until the problem itself is effectively resolved, the person will be dependent on drugs or even addicted to them.

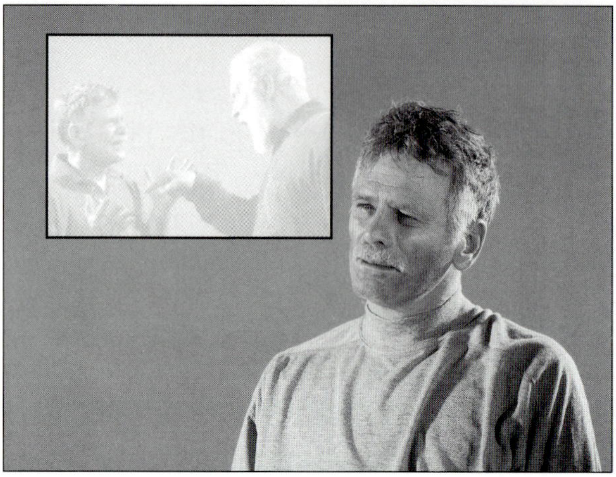

Drugs and Their Effects on the Mind

Drugs essentially are poisons. The degree they are taken determines the effect. A small amount gives a stimulant (increases activity). A greater amount acts as a sedative (suppresses activity). A larger amount acts as a poison and can kill one.

This is true of any drug. Each requires a different amount.

Caffeine is a drug, so coffee is an example. One hundred cups of coffee would probably kill a person. Ten cups would probably put him to sleep. Two or three cups stimulates. This is a very common drug. It is not very harmful as it takes so much of it to have an effect. So it is known as a stimulant.

Arsenic is known as a poison. Yet a tiny amount of arsenic is a stimulant, a good-sized dose puts one to sleep and a few grains kills one.

But there are many drugs which have another liability: they directly affect the mind.

In order to have a good understanding of the mental effects of drugs, it is necessary to know something about what the mind is. The *mind* is not a brain. It is the accumulated recordings of thoughts, conclusions, decisions, observations and perceptions of a person throughout his entire existence. In Scientology it has been discovered that the *mind* is a communication and control system between a thetan and his environment. By *thetan* is meant the person himself, the spiritual being—not his body or his name, the physical universe, his mind, or anything else.

The most obvious portion of the mind is recognizable by anyone not in serious condition. This is the *mental image picture.*

Various phenomena connect themselves with this entity called the mind. Some people closing their eyes see only blackness, some people see pictures.

The mind is a communication and control system between a thetan and his environment. The mind is not a brain.

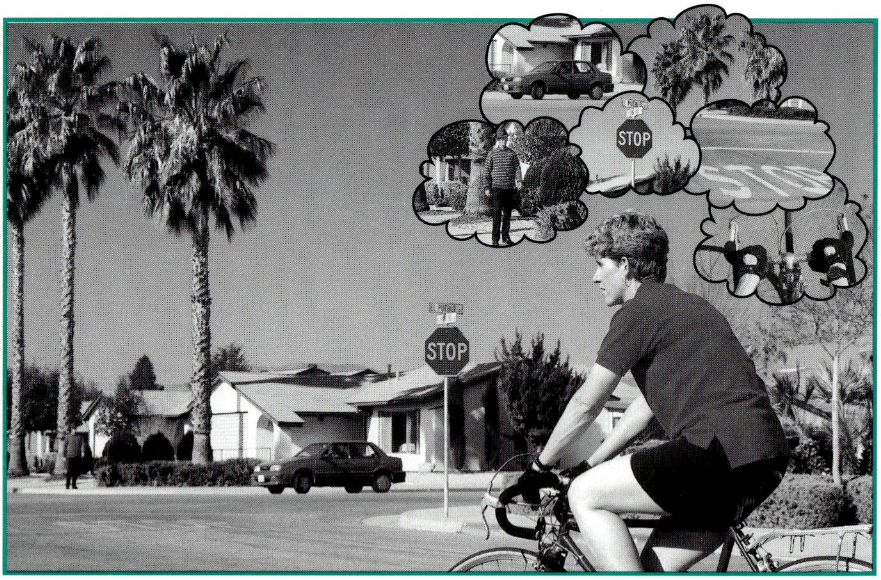

The thetan receives, by the communication system called the mind, various impressions, including direct views of the physical universe. In addition to this he receives impressions from past activities and, most important, he himself conceives things about the past and future which are independent of immediately present stimuli.

A person who has taken drugs, in addition to the physical factors involved, retains mental image pictures of those drugs and their effects. Mental image pictures are three-dimensional color pictures with sound and smell and all other perceptions, plus the conclusions or speculations of the individual. They are mental copies of one's perceptions sometime in the past, although in cases of unconsciousness or lessened consciousness they exist *below* the individual's awareness. For example, a person who had taken LSD would retain "pictures" of that experience in his mind, complete with recordings of the sights, physical sensations, smells, sounds, etc., that occurred while he was under the influence of LSD.

Let us say an individual took LSD one day while at a fairground with some friends, and the day's experiences included feeling nauseated and dizzy, getting into an argument with a friend, feeling an emotion of sadness, and later feeling very tired. He would have mental image pictures of that entire incident.

At a later time, if this person's environment were to contain enough similarities to the elements in that past incident, he may experience a reactivation of that incident. As a result he could feel nauseated, dizzy, sad and very tired—all for no apparent reason. This is known as *restimulation:* the reactivation of a past memory due to similar circumstances in the present approximating circumstances of the past.

Such mental image pictures can also be reactivated by drug residuals, as the presence of these drugs in the tissues of the body can simulate the earlier drug experiences.

Using the above example of the person who took LSD, sometime later—perhaps years afterward—the residuals of the drug that are still in his body tissues can cause a restimulation of that LSD incident. The mental image pictures are reactivated, and he experiences the same sensations of nausea, dizziness and tiredness, and he feels sad. He does not know why. He might also perceive mental images of the persons he was with and the accompanying sights and sounds and smells.

These are the effects on the mind of *past* drug usage. However, the *current* use of drugs creates a similar and more immediate effect on the mind.

When a person uses a drug such as marijuana, peyote, opium, morphine or heroin, mental image pictures of past times can "turn on" or restimulate below the individual's conscious awareness, causing him to perceive something different than what is actually going on.

Thus, right there before your eyes, apparently in the same room as you are, doing the same things, the drug-taker is really only partially there and partially in some past events.

He *seems* to be there. Really he isn't "tracking" fully with present time.

What is going on to a rational observation is *not* what is going on to him.

Thus, he does not understand statements made by another but tries to fit them into his composite reality, meaning a reality made up of different components. In order to fit them in, he has to alter them.

For example, a drug user may be *sure* he is helping one *repair* a

Drugs affect the mind by reactivating incidents from a person's past, below his conscious awareness.

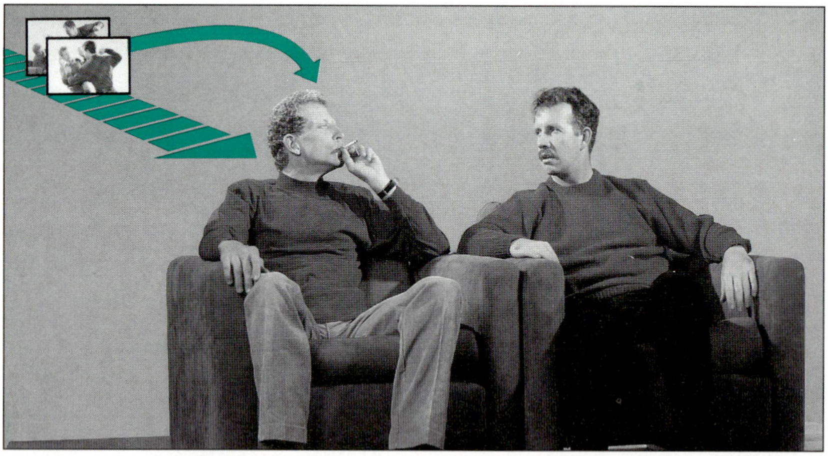

This can distort the drug user's perception of what is happening around him.

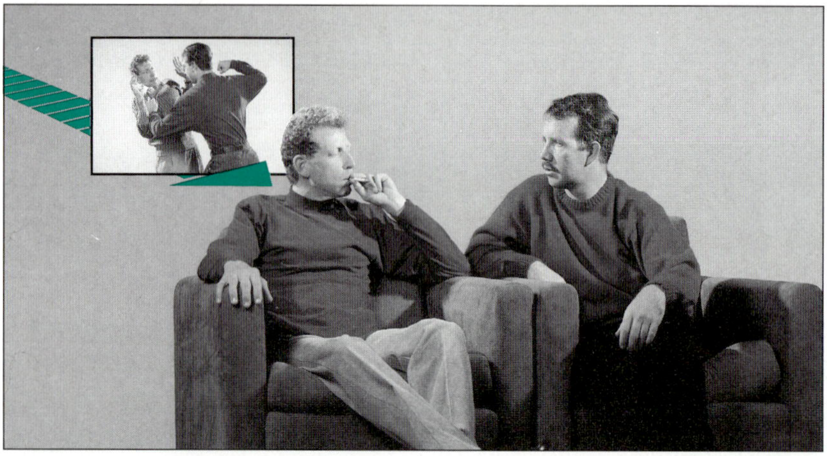

As a result, the person's actions may appear very odd or irrational.

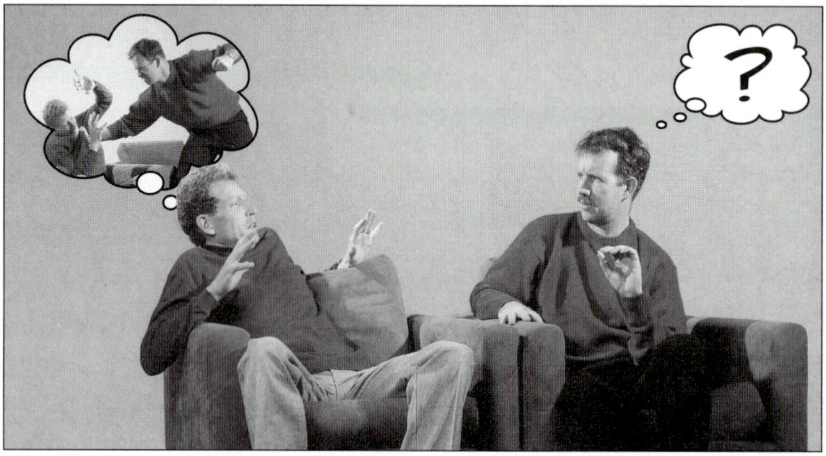

floor that needs fixing, but in fact he is hindering the actual operation in progress which consists of *cleaning* the floor. So when he "helps one" mop the floor, he introduces chaos into the activity. Since *he* is *repairing* the floor, a request to "give me the mop" has to be reinterpreted as "hand me the hammer." But the mop handle is longer than a hammer handle so the bucket gets upset.

This can be slight, wherein the person is seen to make occasional mistakes. It can be as serious as total insanity where the events apparent to him are *completely* different than those apparent to anyone else. And it can be all grades in between.

It is not that he doesn't know what is going on. It is that he perceives *something else* going on instead of the present sequence of events.

Thus, others appear to him to be stupid or unreasonable or insane. As *they* don't agree in their actions and orders with what he *plainly sees* is in progress, "they" aren't sensible. Example: A group is moving furniture. To all but one they are simply moving furniture. This one perceives himself to be "moving geometric shapes into a cloud." Thus, this one "makes mistakes." As the group doesn't see inside him and only sees another like themselves, they can't figure out why he "balls things up so."

Such persons as drug-takers and the insane are thus slightly or wholly on an apparently different time track of "present time" events.

A drug may be taken to drive a person out of an unbearable present time or out of consciousness altogether.

In some persons they do not afterwards return wholly to present time.

A thetan can also escape an unbearable present time by dropping into the past, even without drugs.

The drug-taker and the insane alike have not recovered present time, to a greater or lesser degree. Thus they think they are running on a different time track than they are.

These are the underlying facts in odd human behavior.

As what is going on according to the perception and subjective reality of such a person is varied in greater or lesser degree from the objective reality of others, such a person disturbs the environment and disrupts the smooth running of *any* group—from family to business to nation.

We have all known such a person, so it is not uncommon in the current civilization. The sudden remark which makes no sense, totally out of context with what is being spoken about; the blank stare when given an order or remark—behind these lies a whole imaginary world which is jarred by our attempts to get something done in present time.

The repercussions of drugs then, go far beyond their immediate effects and often influence many others besides the user. The consequences can be very harmful. This is true not only of illegal street drugs but also of medical drugs that are supposed to help people.

Painkillers

Doctors and others prescribe painkillers such as aspirin, tranquilizers, hypnotics and soporifics (sleep-inducing drugs) in an understandable wish to relieve pain.

However, it has never been known in chemistry or medicine exactly how or why these things worked. Such compositions are derived by accidental discoveries that "such and so depresses pain."

The effects of existing compounds are not uniform in result and often have very bad side effects.

As the *reason* they worked was unknown, very little advance has been made in biochemistry—the chemistry of life processes and substances. If the reason they worked were known and accepted, possibly chemists could develop some actual painkillers which had minimal side effects.

Pain or discomfort of a psychosomatic nature comes from mental image pictures created by the thetan which press against and affect the body. For example, a mental image picture of a past incident in which an arm was broken can be reactivated in the present, impinging on the body and causing pain in that same arm.

By actual clinical test, the actions of aspirin and other pain depressants are to:

A. *Inhibit the ability of the thetan to create mental image pictures*

and also

B. *To impede the electrical conductivity of nerve channels.*

As a result, the thetan is rendered *stupid,* blank, forgetful, delusive and irresponsible. He gets into a "wooden" sort of state, unfeeling, insensitive, unable and definitely not trustworthy, a menace to his fellows actually.

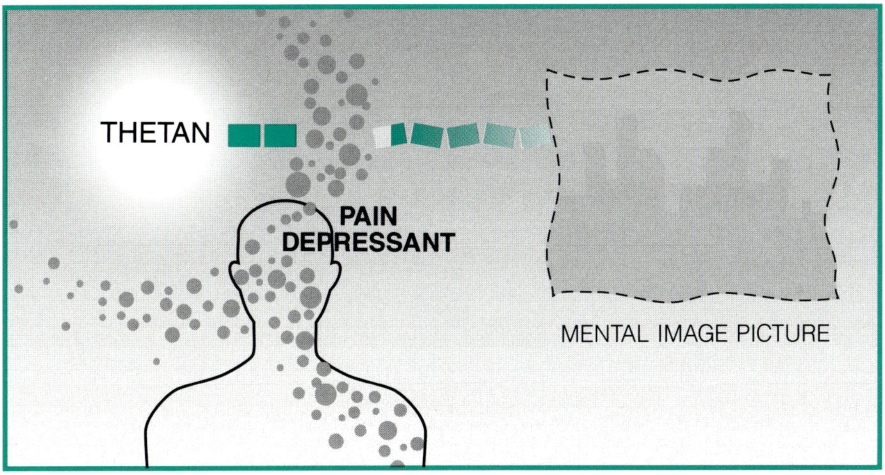

Pain depressants inhibit the thetan's ability to create mental image pictures.

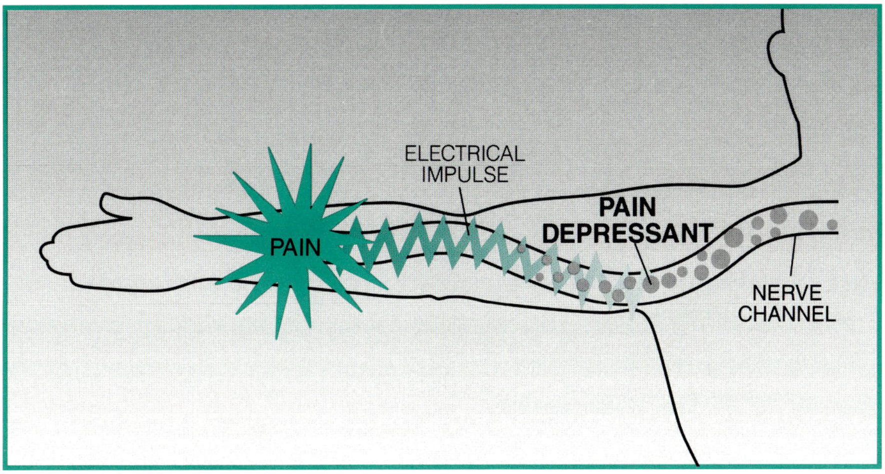

They also act to impede electrical conductivity of the nerve channels.

When the drugs wear off or start to wear off, the ability to create mental image pictures starts to return and *turns on somatics* (body sensations, illnesses or pains or discomforts) *much harder.* One of the answers a person has for this is *more* drugs. To say nothing of heroin, there are aspirin addicts. The compulsion stems from a desire to get rid of the somatics and unwanted sensations again. The being gets more and more wooden, requiring more and more quantity and more frequent use.

Sexually it is common for someone on drugs to be very stimulated at first. But after the original sexual "kicks," the stimulation of sexual sensation becomes harder and harder to achieve. The effort to achieve it becomes obsessive while it itself is less and less satisfying.

The cycle of drug restimulation of pictures (or creation in general) can be at first to increase creation and then eventually inhibit it totally.

If one were working on the problem of pain relief biochemically, the least harmful pain depressant would be one that inhibited the creation of mental image pictures with minimal resulting "woodenness" or stupidity and which was body-soluble (easily dissolved in the body) so that it passed rapidly out of the nerves and system.

There are unwanted sensations that drugs block off, but there is a whole sector of desirable sensations, and drugs block off all sensations.

The only defense that can be made for drugs is that they give a short, quick oblivion from immediate agony and permit the handling of a person to effect repair. But even then this is applicable to persons who have no other system to handle their pain.

Dexterity, ability and alertness are the main things that prevent getting into painful situations. These all vanish with drugs. So drugs set you up to get into situations which are truly disastrous and keep you that way.

One has a choice between being dead with drugs or being alive without them. Drugs rob life of the sensations and joys which are the only reasons for living anyhow.

Helping Someone Get Off Drugs

When the world went into heavy drug abuse, the problem of drying out became one of the first order. All pre-Scientology efforts to help drug users failed—and had been failing throughout man's history.

However, workable solutions have been developed in Scientology which enable a person not only to cease drug use, but to reach and eradicate the root causes which started him or her down that dark road.

Drugs can extract a dreadful price from the user should he ever try to quit.

What is called *withdrawal symptoms* set in. These are the physical and mental reactions to no longer taking drugs. They are ghastly. No torturer ever set up anything worse.

The person had this problem then:

A. Stay on drugs and be trapped and suffering from here on out, or

B. Try to come off the drugs and be so agonizingly ill meanwhile that he couldn't stand it.

This was a dead-if-you-do, dead-if-you-don't sort of problem.

Medicine did not solve it adequately. Psychotherapy was impossible.

Two approaches now exist to this withdrawal problem, both of which should be used:

1. Nutritionist experiments indicate that vitamins and minerals assist the withdrawal.

2. Light Objective Processes ease the gradual withdrawal and make it possible.

A *process* is an exact series of directions or sequence of actions taken to accomplish a desired result. Its application is called *processing.* There are many processes contained in the materials of Scientology which can be used to help a person direct his attention off himself and onto his environment and the people and things in it—an action which is very therapeutic for someone coming off drugs. These are called Objective Processes. When properly used, they ease the person's symptoms and make drug withdrawal possible with a minimum of discomfort.

Objective refers to outward things, not the thoughts or feelings of the individual. *Objective Processes* deal with the real and observable. They call for the person to spot or find something exterior to himself in order to carry out the procedures.

The Objective Processes referred to here are called "light" Objective Processes in that they are simpler and less advanced than other Objective Processes which exist in Scientology.

The details of how to use these two approaches to getting someone unhooked from drugs follow. If you know someone who is dependent on drugs, you can help him withdraw from them by applying the principles and techniques given here.

On severe cases of drug addiction one should send the person to a qualified medical doctor for examination to determine if there are any special precautions that may need to be taken for that particular person.

Some persons may have been put on some therapeutic drug by a medical doctor and possibly should remain on it. But these are not the usual drugs we are dealing with. It is up to the person and the doctor what should be done in such cases.

Nutritional Data

According to world-renowned nutritionist Adelle Davis, vitamin therapy has had success in handling withdrawal symptoms.

Instead of just telling the person to break off drugs with all that suffering and danger of failure, the patient is given heavy doses of vitamins. The data is repeated here for information.

The Drug Bomb

A vitamin formula called the "drug bomb" has been found effective in combating the effects of withdrawal. It consists of:

1,000 milligrams of niacinamide (*not* nicotinic acid). This helps counteract any mental disturbance.

5,000 IU of vitamin A.

400 IU of vitamin D.

800 IU of vitamin E.

2,000 milligrams of vitamin C.

500 milligrams of magnesium carbonate (to make the vitamin C effective).

25 milligrams of B_6.

200 milligrams of B complex.

300 milligrams of B_1.

100 milligrams of pantothenic acid.

This formula should be given four times a day while a person is coming off drugs, roughly every six hours.

It should *not* be taken on an empty stomach, as it could cause stomach burn. It should be taken after meals or, if taken between meals, with yogurt.

Great caution must be taken to give the dose in such a way that the vitamins will not corrode the stomach. If this is neglected, the person can be given a false duodenal (upper intestine) ulcer and will be unable to continue the treatment. Drug users are usually in terrible physical condition anyway. Thus, the vitamins would have to be in "enteric coated" tablets, meaning an intestinal shielding must be on the pills so they gradually dissolve and don't hit the sensitive upper stomach hard enough to corrode it.

Thus, milk with powdered amino acids in it would have to be given to wash the pills down.

In testing these recommendations, stomach corrosion (wearing away) from the vitamin formula was the main barrier noted.

If the formula is given without any cushion, the person can (a) feel too full after eating, (b) have a stomachache, (c) have a burning sensation, (d) the exterior of the stomach can get sore. These are all stomach ulcer symptoms.

If such symptoms turn on, end off the vitamins. Aluminum hydroxide tablets chewed up and swallowed in milk each time the symptoms start will ease the stomach. Powdered amino acids, yogurt and milk must then be given until the stomach gets better.

The potential benefits of the drug bomb far outweigh any possible drawbacks and so it has much value. The difficulties and agonies of withdrawal are the primary failure point in trying to salvage a being from the insanity of drugs.

Calcium and Magnesium

Used in conjunction with the drug bomb, there is an additional method of alleviating drug withdrawal symptoms which involves use of the minerals calcium and magnesium.

Muscular spasms are caused by lack of calcium. Nervous reactions are diminished by magnesium.

Calcium does not go into solution in the body and is not utilized unless it is in an acid.

Tests for other uses than drug reactions brought about the means of getting calcium into solution in the body along with magnesium so that the results of both could be achieved. The answer was to add vinegar, which would provide the acidic formula needed.

The result was a solution which proved to be highly effective, named the "Cal-Mag Formula."

The use of Cal-Mag, experimental in the early 1970s to help ease withdrawal symptoms, is now long past the experimental stage. Cal-Mag has been used very effectively during withdrawal to help ease and counteract the convulsions, muscular spasms and severe nervous reactions experienced by an addict when coming off drugs.

The Cal-Mag Formula uses a ratio of one part elemental magnesium to two parts elemental calcium, mixed with vinegar in water.

As the formula calls for precise amounts of calcium and magnesium, some further explanation of these quantities should be given here.

The Cal-Mag Formula is made using the compounds calcium gluconate and magnesium carbonate. Both of these come in white, powdery form. Each is a compound of different substances. In other words, calcium gluconate contains other substances besides calcium; it is not all pure calcium but contains only a percentage of pure elemental calcium. Similarly, magnesium carbonate contains other substances besides magnesium, and includes only a percentage of pure elemental magnesium.

But it is the amount of elemental magnesium in correct ratio to the amount of elemental calcium that is important in the preparation of the Cal-Mag Formula. This does *not* mean that you use pure magnesium or pure calcium when you make Cal-Mag. Use only calcium gluconate and magnesium carbonate.

Magnesium Carbonate: The desired compound for Cal-Mag, called magnesium carbonate basic, contains 29 percent magnesium. (This compound is also sometimes called magnesium alba.)

There are different magnesium compounds with different percentages of elemental magnesium, but using any kind other than that recommended here will give varying amounts of magnesium which will violate the needed ratio of one part magnesium to two parts calcium.

It is magnesium carbonate basic, containing 29 percent elemental magnesium which is used in making Cal-Mag. And it is essential to ensure that the magnesium carbonate basic which is used is fresh, not old.

Calcium Gluconate: There is only one kind of calcium gluconate compound and nine percent of that compound is calcium, so there is no problem in selecting the correct calcium gluconate compound for the Cal-Mag preparation.

The ingredients can be obtained in most health food stores or where vitamins are sold.

To prepare Cal-Mag:

1. Put one level tablespoon (15 ml) of calcium gluconate in a normal-sized glass.

2. Add ½ level teaspoon (2.5 ml) of magnesium carbonate.

3. Add 1 tablespoon (15 ml) of cider vinegar (at least 5 percent acidity).

4. Stir it well.

5. Add ½ glass (about 120 ml) of boiling water and stir until all the powder is dissolved and the liquid is clear. (If this doesn't occur it could be from poor grade or old magnesium carbonate.)

6. Fill the remainder of glass with lukewarm or cold water and cover.

You can make larger quantities at one time, simply by multiplying all the ingredients accordingly. The solution will stay good for two days.

It can be made wrongly so that it does not dissolve. Variations from the above produce an unsuccessful mix that can taste pretty horrible.

(Note, again, that the ratio is one part elemental magnesium to two parts elemental calcium. If one wants to work this out precisely, one can work out the elemental amounts. The formula above has been given for the compound amounts.)

Anything from one to three glasses of this a day, with or after meals, *replaces any tranquilizer.* It does not produce the drugged effects of tranquilizers (which are quite deadly).

It has proven effective in helping to handle the muscular spasms, tics and nervous reactions that can occur as a result of drug withdrawal.

It should be mentioned that many health food stores do carry premixed preparations of calcium and magnesium. Before using any of these in place of Cal-Mag, one should read the label to see if the calcium and magnesium are given in correct proportions and check if it contains acid (such as ascorbic acid or citric acid). Otherwise, such preparations are worthless and will not give the same results as the Cal-Mag Formula.

How to Prepare Cal-Mag

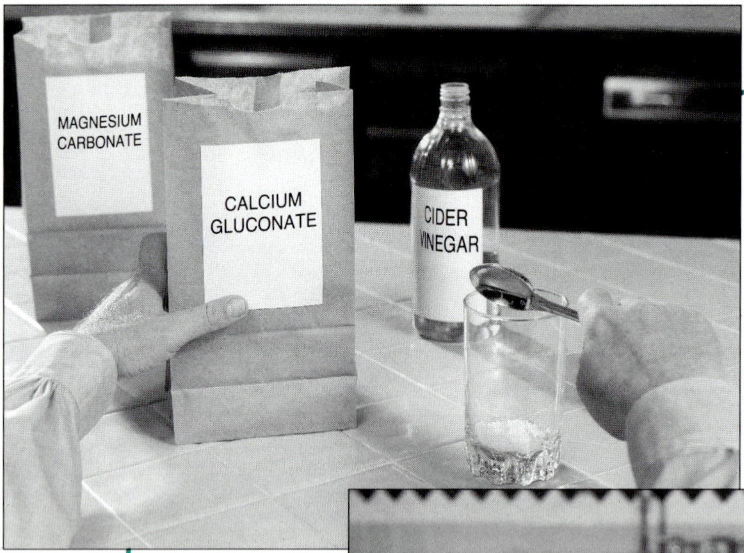

1. Put 1 level tablespoon (15 ml) of calcium gluconate in a normal-sized glass. Use a measuring spoon, not tableware.

2. Add ½ level teaspoon (2.5 ml) of magnesium carbonate. Again, use a proper measuring spoon.

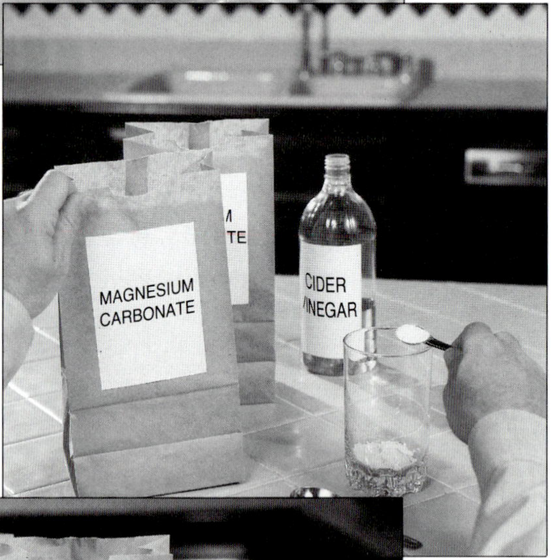

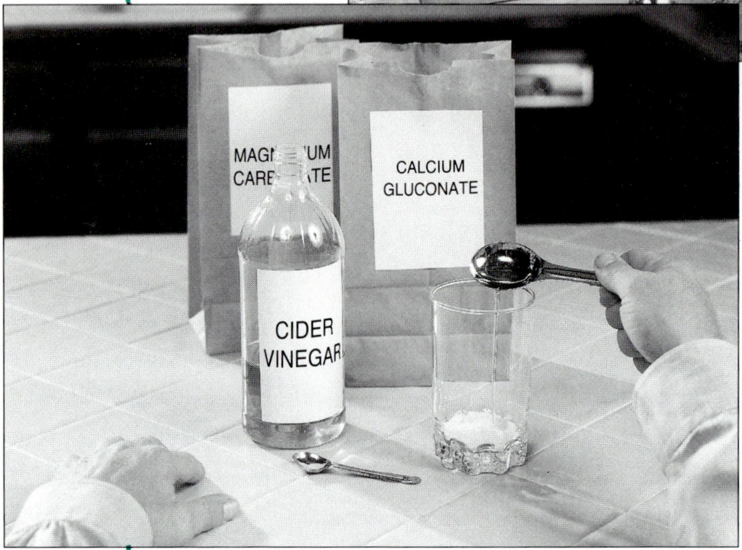

3. Add 1 tablespoon (15 ml) cider vinegar (at least 5 percent acidity).

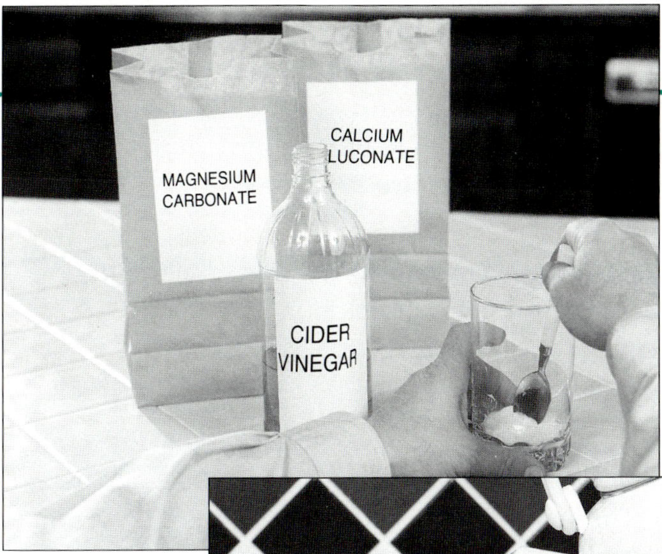

4. Stir it well.

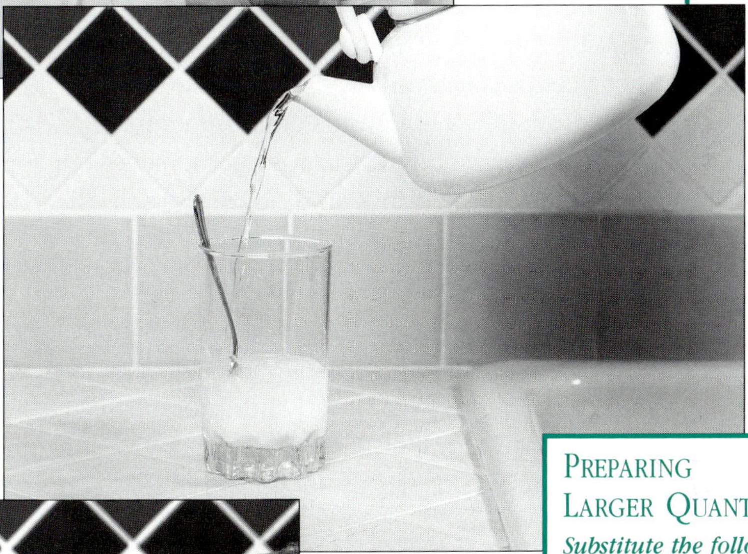

5. Add ½ glass (about 120 ml) of boiling water and stir until all the powder is dissolved and the liquid is clear. (Note: Place a metal spoon in the glass first to avoid any possibility of the glass cracking from the boiling water.)

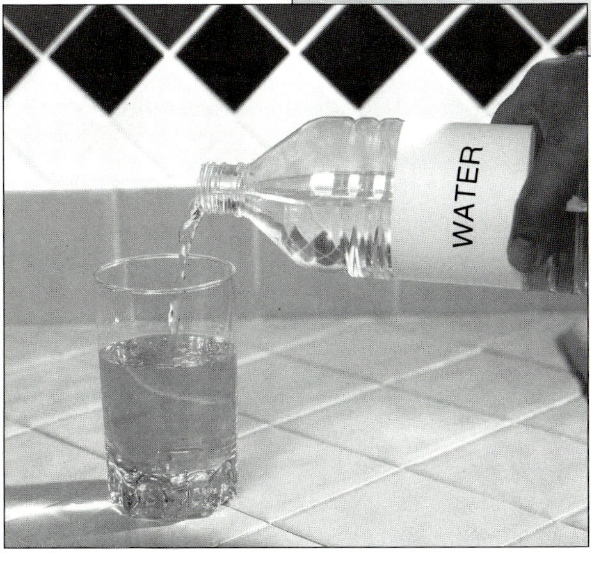

6. Fill the remainder of glass with lukewarm or cold water.

Preparing Larger Quantities

Substitute the following quantities in the formula to make 1 gallon (approx. 4 liters) of Cal-Mag:

A. 13 tablespoons (195 ml) calcium gluconate

B. 6.5 teaspoons (33 ml) magnesium carbonate

C. 6.5 ounces (195 ml) cider vinegar

D. ½ gallon (approx. 2 liters) boiling water

Fill the remainder with lukewarm or cold water.

Objective Processes

In addition to nutritional handling, the other approach to the drug withdrawal problem consists of Objective Processes.

Because drugs tend to push a person into experiences of the past and stick his attention in these moments, processes which pull more of a person's attention outward help unstick him from the past.

There are many Objective Processes in Scientology which accomplish this.

Objective Processes help a person get into present time and become more aware of his surroundings and other people and away from past problems. The more a person is able to face the present, and not be stuck in the past, the more he can enjoy life. He can be in better communication with his environment as it exists, not as it once was. This is worthwhile for anyone to achieve, but for someone who has been heavily on drugs and suffered their ill effects it can be a revelation.

Five Objective Processes are included here.

It is best to do these processes in a quiet place, free of distraction or interruption and with enough time to do the process until the person being helped has good indicators and has had a cognition. *Indicators* are conditions or circumstances arising during a process which indicate (point out or show) whether it is going well or badly. The person looking brighter or more cheerful, for example, has good indicators. A *cognition* is a new realization about life. It is a "What do you know, I . . ." statement; something a person suddenly understands or feels.

These processes are given to the person in addition to the drug bomb and Cal-Mag. They are very effective when given several times a day to help get the person through the period of withdrawal from drugs, which usually takes about a week or less. For example, a person could be given one of these processes in the morning, and some hours later he could be given another. A person going through withdrawal often sleeps considerably more than usual, especially at the beginning of such a program. Therefore, one would not go at this too strenuously; giving the person two or three of these Objective Processes each day should be sufficient to get a result.

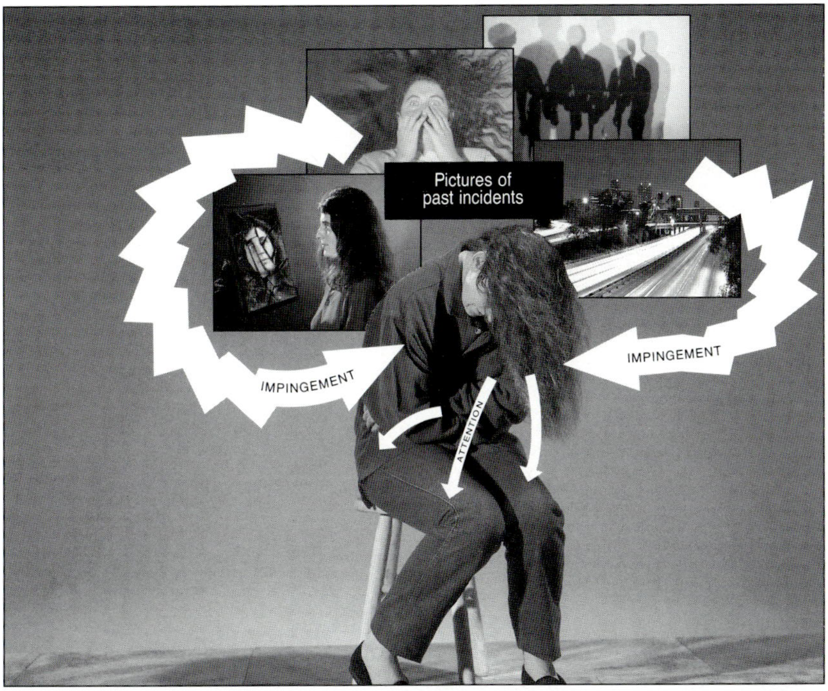

The attention of a person withdrawing from drug use can be very stuck on the body, and past incidents can be reactivated heavily.

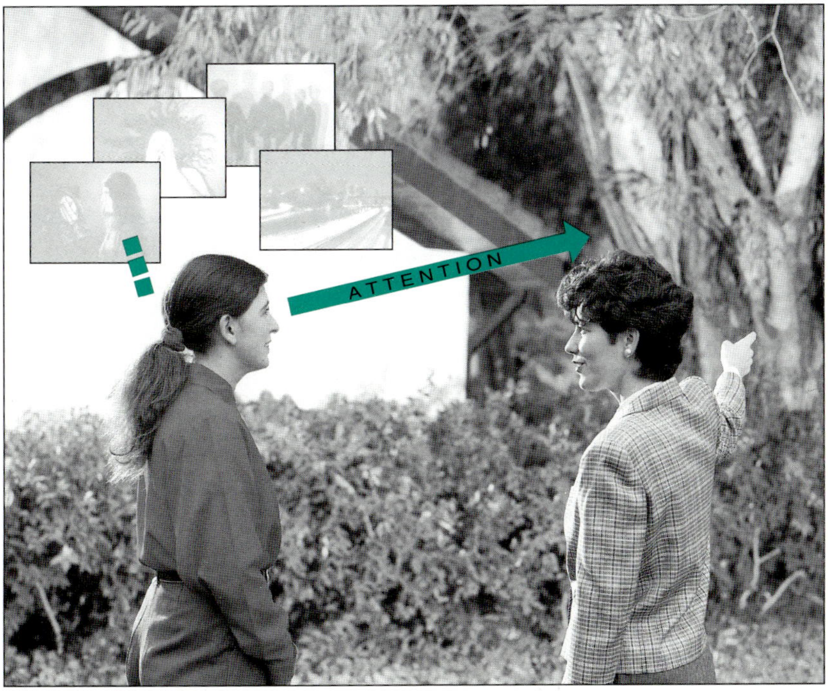

Light Objective Processes can extrovert the person's attention and greatly ease any discomfort. Past incidents drop out of the present and no longer impinge on the person.

"Notice That"

This process directs a person's attention off his body and out onto the environment. The procedure is as follows:

1. Tell the person you are going to process him and briefly explain the procedure.

2. The command used is:

"Notice that __________ (indicated object)."

Ensure he understands it.

3. Indicate an obvious object by pointing to it. Tell the person, "Notice that __________ (object)."

4. When the person has done so, acknowledge him by saying, "Thank you" or "Okay" or "Good," etc.

5. Continue giving the command, directing the person's attention to different objects in the environment. Be sure to acknowledge the person each time after he has carried out the command.

For example, say:

"Notice that chair."

"Thank you."

"Notice that window."

"All right."

"Notice that floor."

"Very good."

And so on.

6. Continue the process until the person being helped has good indicators and has had a cognition.

You can end the process at this point. Tell the person, "End of process."

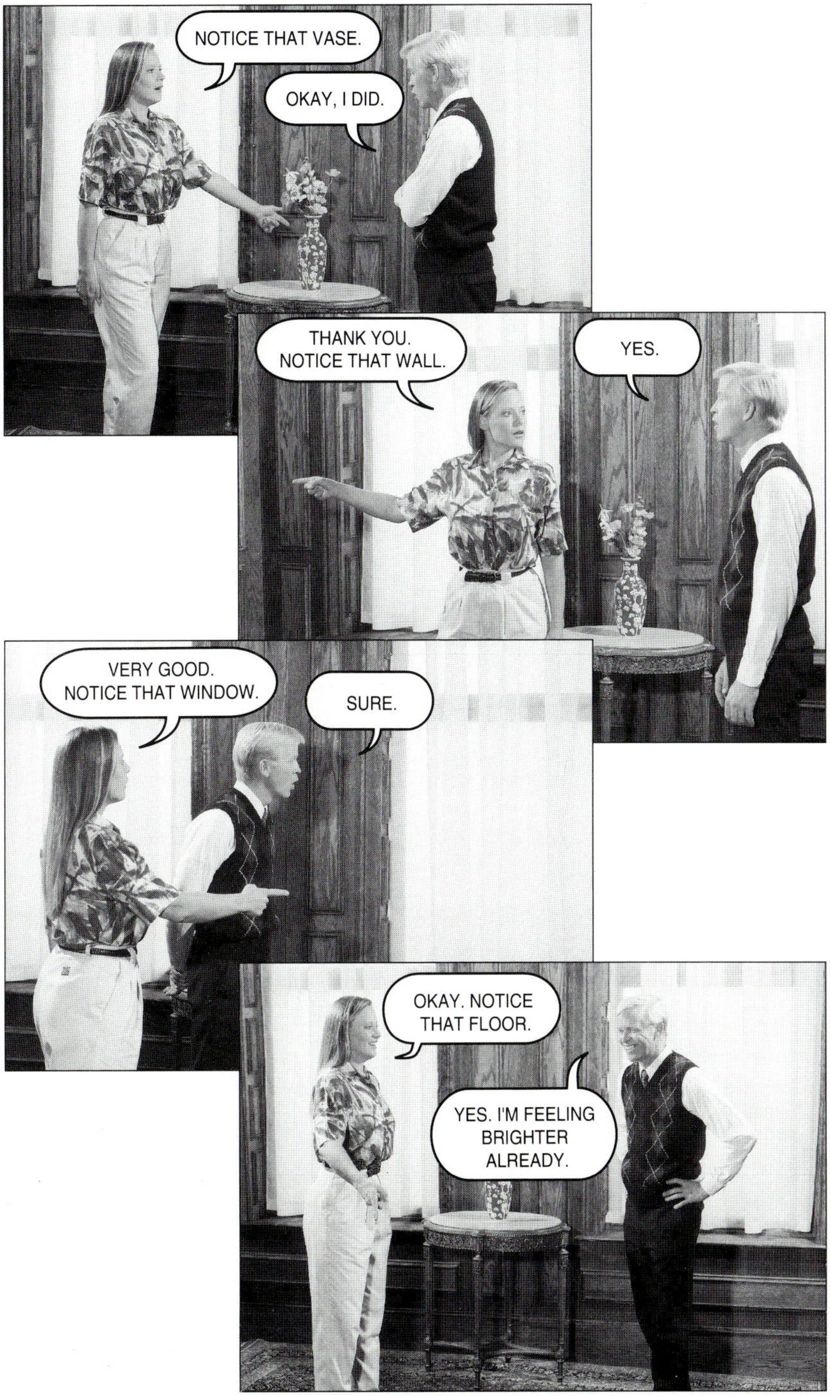
NOTICE THAT VASE.
OKAY, I DID.
THANK YOU. NOTICE THAT WALL.
YES.
VERY GOOD. NOTICE THAT WINDOW.
SURE.
OKAY. NOTICE THAT FLOOR.
YES. I'M FEELING BRIGHTER ALREADY.

A Havingness Process

Havingness is the feeling that one owns or possesses. It can also be described as the concept of being able to reach or not being prevented from reaching. This process puts a person's attention onto the environment so he can have it. The procedure is as follows:

1. Tell the person you are going to process him and briefly explain the procedure.

2. The command used is:

"Look around here and find something you could have."

Ensure he understands it.

3. Give the command, "Look around here and find something you could have."

4. When the person has done so, acknowledge him by saying, "Thank you" or "Okay" or "Good," etc.

5. Continue giving the command. Be sure to acknowledge the person each time after he has carried out the command.

For example, say:

"Look around here and find something you could have."

"Thank you."

"Look around here and find something you could have."

"Good."

"Look around here and find something you could have."

"All right."

"Look around here and find something you could have."

"Very good."

And so on.

6. Continue the process until the person being helped has good indicators and has had a cognition. You end the process at this point. Tell the person, "End of process."

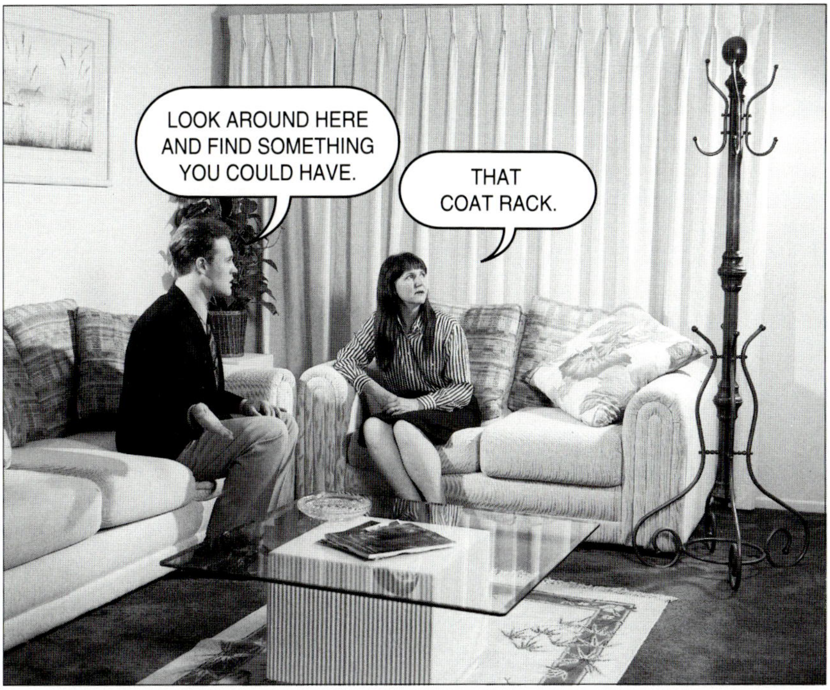
LOOK AROUND HERE AND FIND SOMETHING YOU COULD HAVE.
THAT COAT RACK.

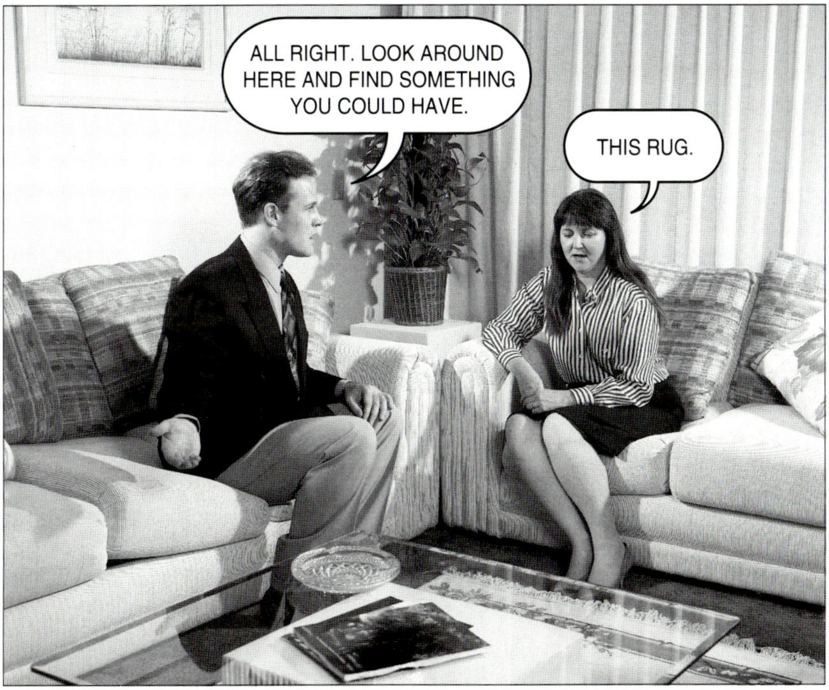
ALL RIGHT. LOOK AROUND HERE AND FIND SOMETHING YOU COULD HAVE.
THIS RUG.

"Touch That"

This process is done with both persons walking about, or if the person being helped is not able to walk, they may be seated at a table with a number of objects scattered on its surface. The procedure is as follows:

1. Tell the person you are going to process him and briefly explain the procedure.

2. The command used is:

"Touch that __________ (indicated object)."

Choose different objects in the room for the person to touch.

Ensure the person understands the command.

3. Give the command, "Touch that __________ (indicated object)."

4. When the person has done so, acknowledge him.

5. Continue giving the command. Be sure to acknowledge the person each time after he has carried out the command.

For example, say:

"Touch that table."

"Thank you."

"Touch that chair."

"Good."

And so on.

6. Continue the process until the person being helped has good indicators and has had a cognition. You end the process at this point. Tell the person, "End of process."

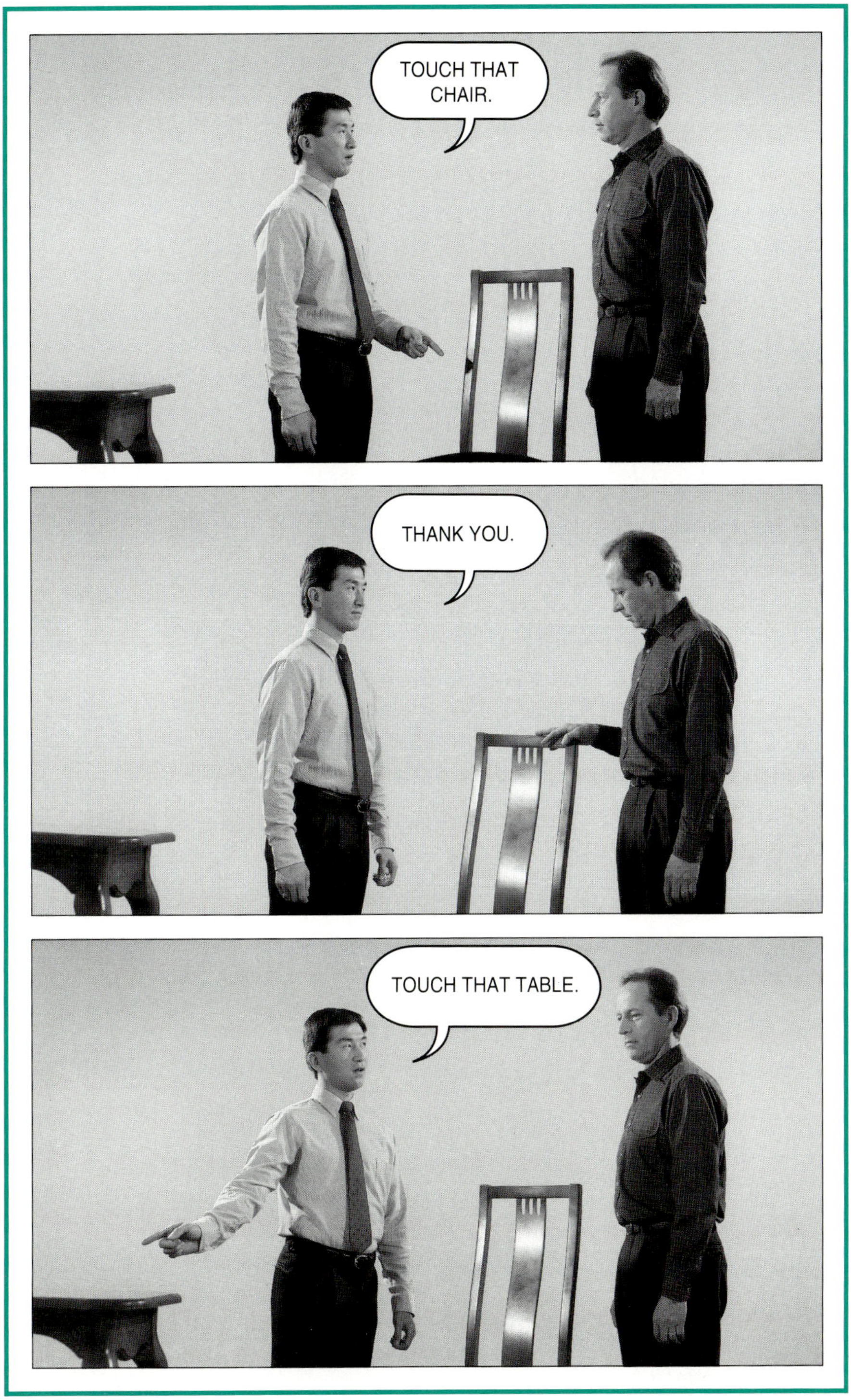
TOUCH THAT CHAIR.
THANK YOU.
TOUCH THAT TABLE.

Touch and Let Go on Room Objects

This is a very good technique and will raise the person's reality on the objects in the room. The procedure is as follows:

1. Tell the person you are going to process him and briefly explain the procedure.

2. The commands used are:

a. "What in the room is really real to you?"

b. "Go over and touch it."

c. "Now let go of it."

Ensure he understands them.

3. Give the command, "What in the room is really real to you?"

4. When the person has answered, acknowledge him.

5. Then give the next command, "Go over and touch it."

6. When the person has done so, acknowledge him.

7. Then give the next command, "Now let go of it."

8. When the person has done so, acknowledge him.

9. Continue giving the commands in this sequence: a, b, c, a, b, c, etc. Be sure to acknowledge the person each time after he has carried out the command.

For example, say:

"What in the room is really real to you?"

"Thank you."

"Go over and touch it."

"Good."

"Now let go of it."

"All right."

"What in the room is really real to you?"

"Very good."

And so on.

10. Continue the process until the person being helped has good indicators and has had a cognition. You end the process at this point. Tell the person, "End of process."

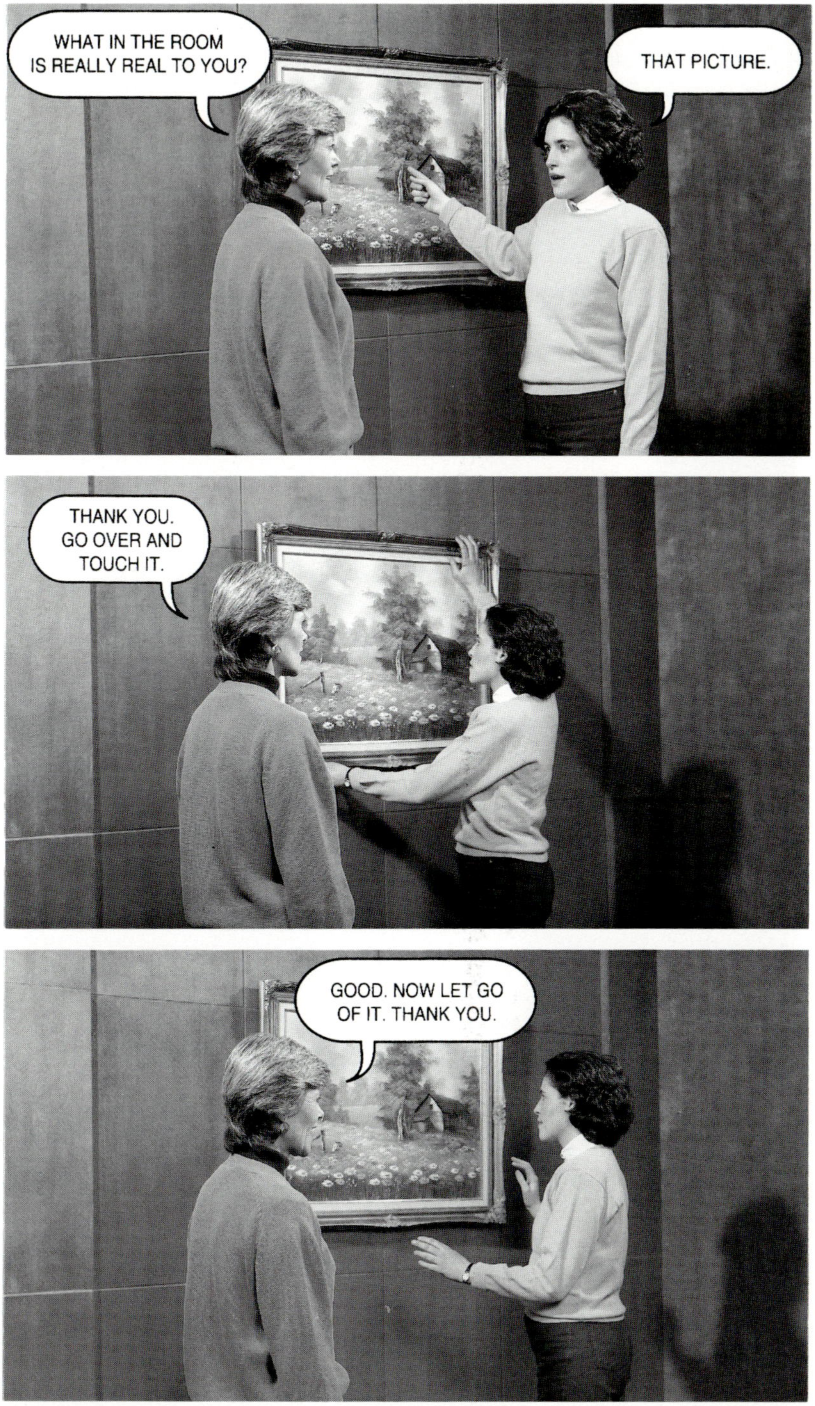
WHAT IN THE ROOM IS REALLY REAL TO YOU?
THAT PICTURE.
THANK YOU. GO OVER AND TOUCH IT.
GOOD. NOW LET GO OF IT. THANK YOU.

"Become Curious About That"

This is a basic Objective Process and is very simple. The procedure is as follows:

1. Tell the person you are going to process him and briefly explain the procedure.

2. The command used is:

"Become curious about that."

Ensure he understands it.

3. Indicate an object in the room by pointing at it and say, "Become curious about that."

You don't call the object by name, you just indicate it. You *don't* say, "Become curious about that chair."

4. When the person has done so, acknowledge him by saying, "Thank you" or "Okay" or "Good," etc.

5. Continue the procedure giving the command. Be sure to acknowledge the person each time after he has carried out the command.

For example, say:

"Become curious about that." (Indicate an object.)

"Thank you."

"Become curious about that." (Indicate an object.)

"Good."

"Become curious about that." (Indicate an object.)

"All right."

"Become curious about that." (Indicate an object.)

"Very good."

And so on.

6. Continue the process until the person being helped has good indicators and has had a cognition. You end the process at this point. Tell the person, "End of process."

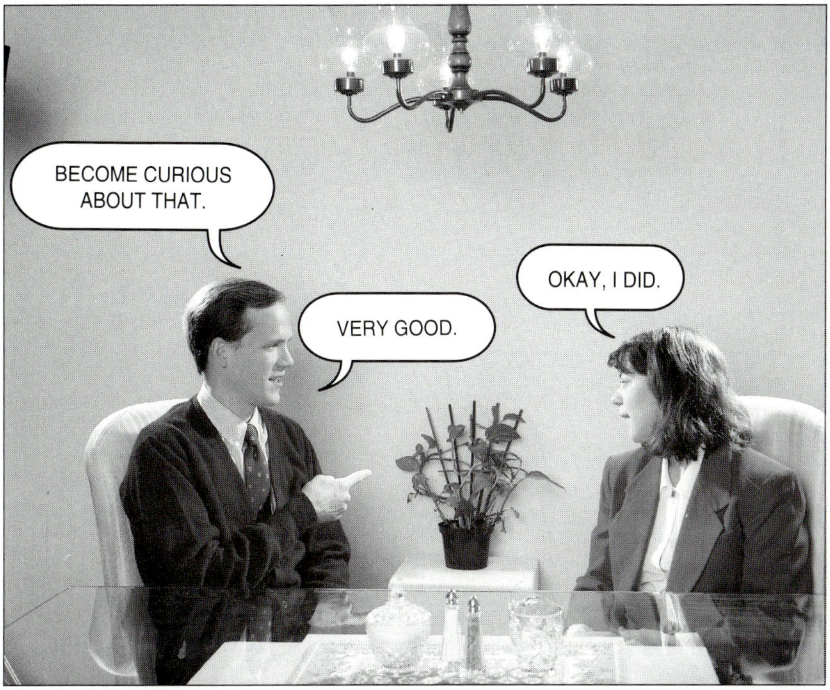
BECOME CURIOUS ABOUT THAT.
VERY GOOD.
OKAY, I DID.

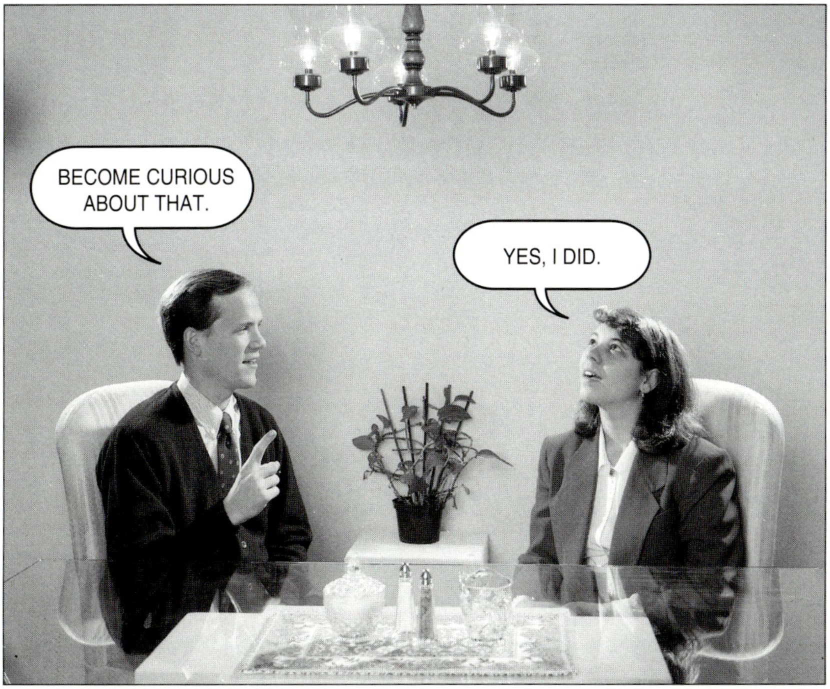
BECOME CURIOUS ABOUT THAT.
YES, I DID.

The Full Resolution

Once a person has been gotten off drugs, other factors must be addressed in order to achieve a full recovery.

This applies to any former drug user, whether the person has recently withdrawn from drugs or stopped using them years earlier. It applies to persons who were never "hard drug users" as well as those who were.

The Purification Program

We live in a chemical-oriented society. One would be hard put to find someone in the present-day civilization who is not affected by this fact. The vast majority of the public is subjected every day to the intake of food preservatives and other chemical poisons including atmospheric poisons, pesticides and the like. Added to this are the pain pills, tranquilizers and other medical drugs used and prescribed by doctors. And we have as well the widespread use of marijuana, LSD, angel dust and other street drugs which contribute heavily to the scene.

In 1977, L. Ron Hubbard discovered that LSD apparently stays in the system for years after the person took it, lodging in the tissues—mainly the fatty tissues of the body—and is liable to go into action again, giving the person unpredictable "trips."

The "restimulation" experienced by people who had been on LSD appeared to act as if they had just taken more LSD.

From subsequent research it appears that not only LSD but other chemical poisons and toxic substances, preservatives and pesticides, as well as medical drugs and the long list of heavy street drugs (angel dust, heroin, marijuana, etc.) can lodge in the tissues and remain in the body for years.

Even medicinal drugs such as diet pills, codeine, Novocain and others have gone into restimulation years after they were taken and had supposedly been eliminated from the body.

Thus it seems that any or all of these hostile biochemical substances can get caught up in the tissues and their accumulation probably disarranges the biochemistry and fluid balance of the body.

The consequences are numerous. Tests show that the learning rate of a person who has been on drugs is much lower than a nondrug person. And the memory of a person who has been on drugs is such as to remove him from fear of consequences.

The being (thetan) of course has mental image pictures of these toxic substances and as long as those substances are in the body, they can restimulate a being. When they are gone from the body, the constant restimulation can cease. So it is actually a spiritual action that is being done.

In Scientology, we have an effective method to cleanse the body of these substances; it is called the Purification program, and it will benefit anyone who lives in this society so inundated with toxins and chemicals.

The Purification program is a tightly supervised regimen which includes:

Exercise

Sauna sweat-out

Nutrition, including vitamins, minerals, etc., as well as oil intake

A properly ordered personal schedule

Exercise: The exercise on this program is in the form of running. The purpose of this is *not* to generate sweat but to get the blood circulating and the system functioning so that impurities held in the system can be released and are pumped out.

Sauna sweat-out: Following the running, the person goes into the sauna to sweat. The impurities can now be dispelled from the body and leave the system through the pores.

Nutrition (including vitamins, minerals and oil intake): When we speak of nutrition we are not talking only about food, but about vitamins and minerals as well, as these are vital to proper nutrition and vital to the effectiveness of this program. We are not, however, talking about "diet" in the overused sense of the word. The person simply eats what he normally eats. He should make sure he gets some vegetables and that the vegetables aren't overcooked.

Toxic substances tend to lock up *mainly,* but not exclusively, in the fat tissue of the body. The theory, then, is that one could replace the fat tissues that hold these toxic accumulations. The body will actually tend to hold on to something it is short of. Thus, if you try to get rid of something it is short of, it won't give it up. So, in the matter of oil, if the person takes some oil, the body might possibly exchange the good oil for the bad fat in the body. That is the basic theory. There are particular vegetable oils which are used for this purpose.

One of the things that toxins and drugs do is create nutritional deficiencies in the body in the form of vitamin and mineral deficiencies. It is easily seen that there is a wide range of toxic substances which create nutritional deficiencies. Alcohol, for example, depends for its effects on a person being able to burn up vitamin B_1. When it burns up all the B_1 in the system the person goes into dt's (delirium tremens) and nightmares.

In the case of other toxic substances the probability exists that other vitamins besides B_1 are burned up. What we seem to have hit on here is that the LSD and street drugs burn up not only B_1 and B complex (which we assume they do) but also create a deficiency in niacin in the body and that they possibly depend on niacin (one of the B complex vitamins) for their effect.

Niacin is essential to nutrition and vital to the effectiveness of the Purification program. It can produce some startling and, in the end, very beneficial results when taken properly on the program, along with the other necessary vitamins and minerals in sufficient and proportionate quantities and along with proper running and sweat-out. Taken in sufficient quantities it appears to break up and unleash LSD, marijuana and other drugs and poisons from the tissues and cells. It can rapidly release LSD crystals into the system. Running and sweating must be done in conjunction with taking niacin to ensure the toxic substances it releases actually do get flushed out of the body.

A properly ordered personal schedule: It is important that a person on this program maintains a properly ordered personal schedule. This means that once one has started on the program he must stick to it sensibly and not skip days or do it in a random fashion. It also means that one should get enough sleep. If one proceeds through the program in an orderly fashion it will be faster and more effective.

The Purification program does not supplant the actions described earlier in this booklet for persons currently on drugs who are apt to experience withdrawal symptoms when taken off of them. The program would be begun only after such technology was applied.

The Harmful Effects of Drugs

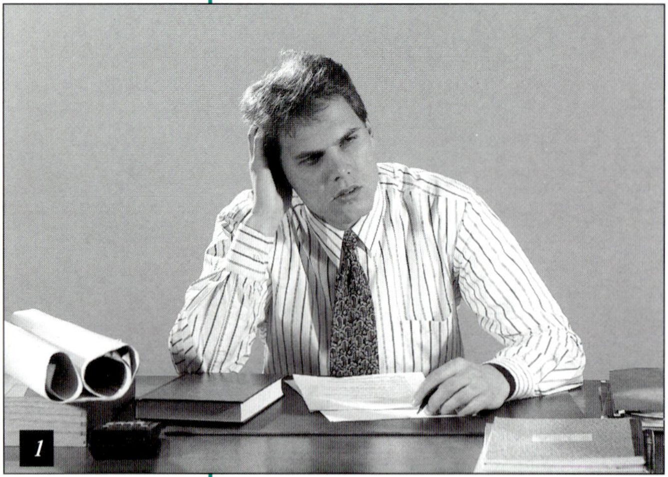

In a drug-ridden world, the individual often finds himself victimized by the harmful effects of drugs, medicine and alcohol, even if taken years before.

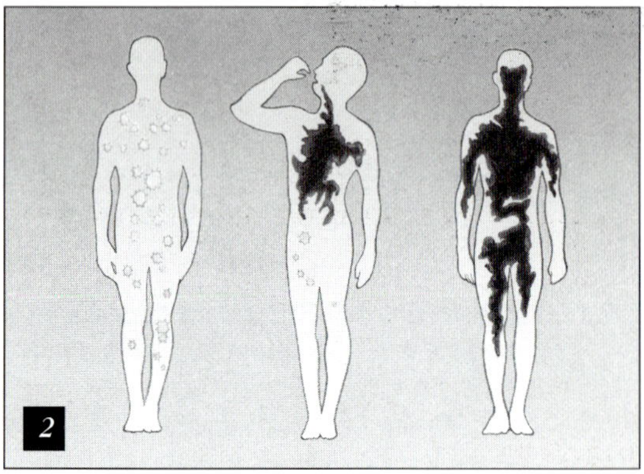

Drugs are essentially poisons and take their toll on a person's body by eating up its stores of vitamins and minerals.

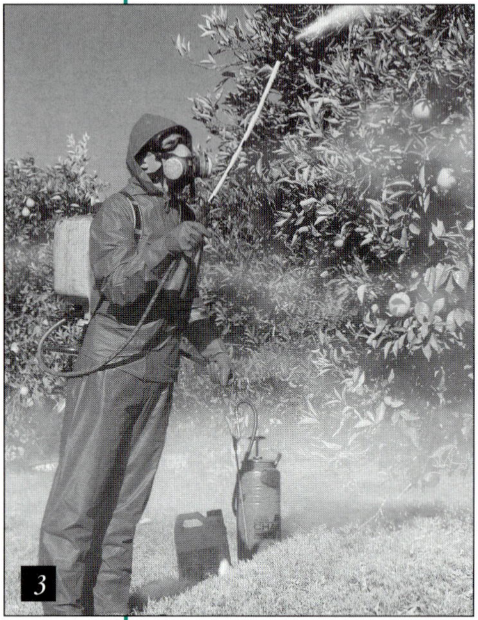

Besides drugs, our world is awash with other substances toxic to human life.

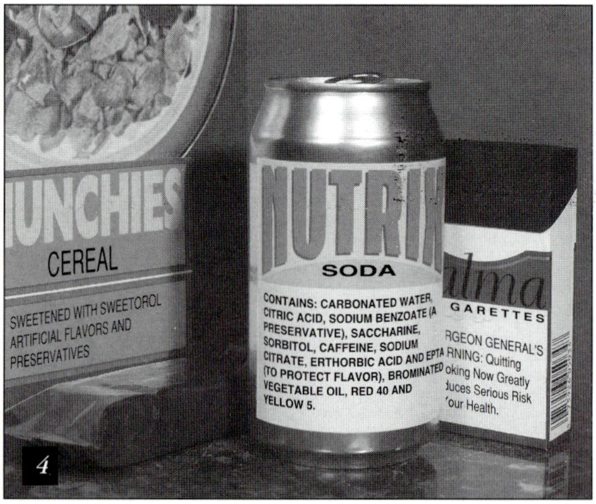

There are literally thousands of artificial substances around that can enter a person's system, many of which are toxic. We live in a chemical-oriented society.

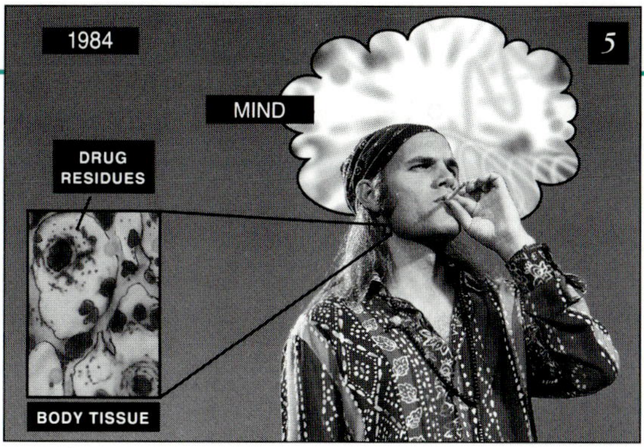

It is a proven fact that drug residues can be trapped in the body.

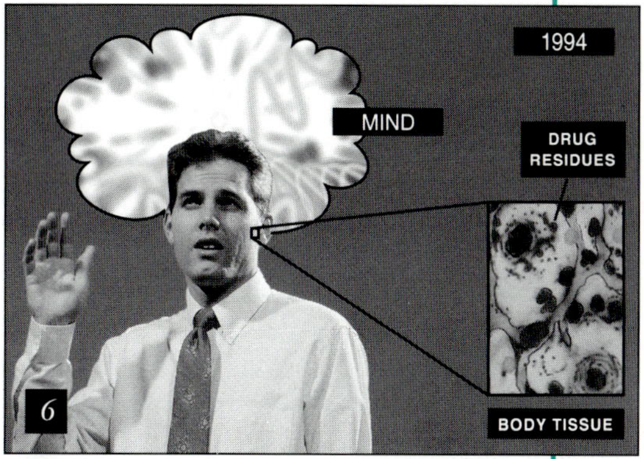

Years later, these residues can dislodge and begin to affect the person again.

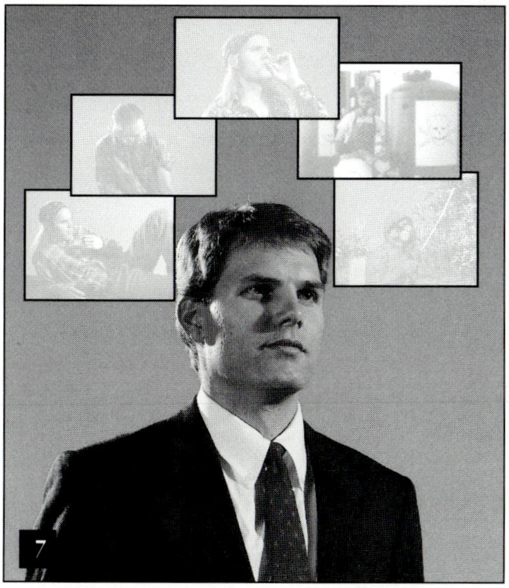

Though a person is no longer taking drugs, he has mental pictures of drugs and drug experiences . . .

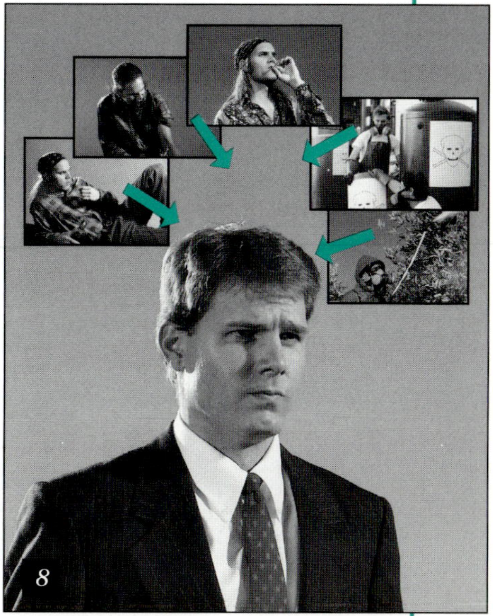

. . . which can reactivate as long as toxic drug residues are locked in the body. A person's awareness, ability and attitudes can be adversely affected.

The Purification Program Illustrated

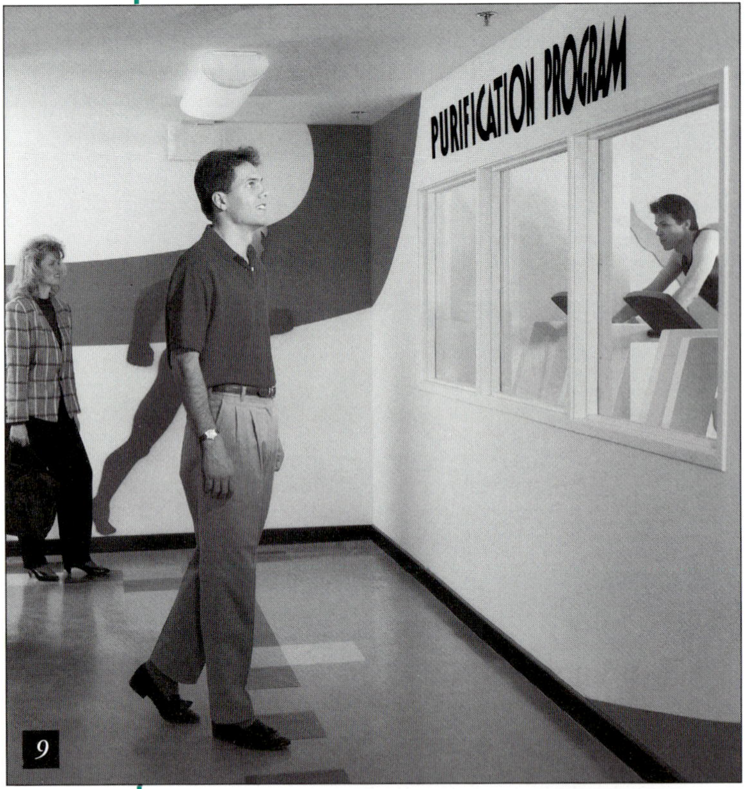

9

There is however a way out of this trap: the Purification program, an exact regimen which can rid the body of harmful drug residues and other toxic substances.

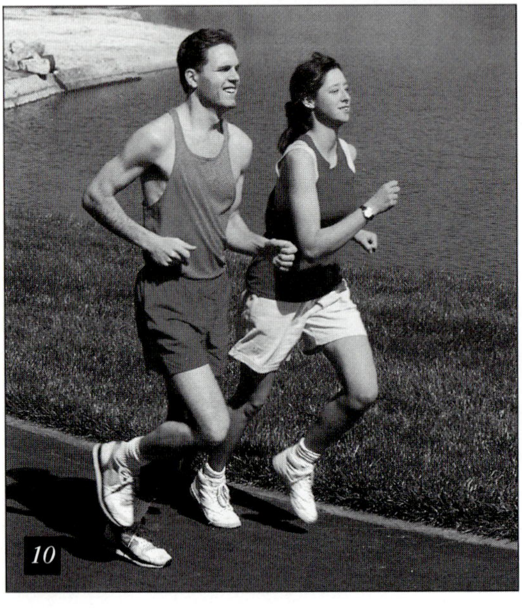
10

After a medical checkup and orientation to the program, a person runs for a period to g the blood circulating faster and the system warmed up.

Increased circulation goes deeper into tissues where harmful deposits are trapped and dislodges them.

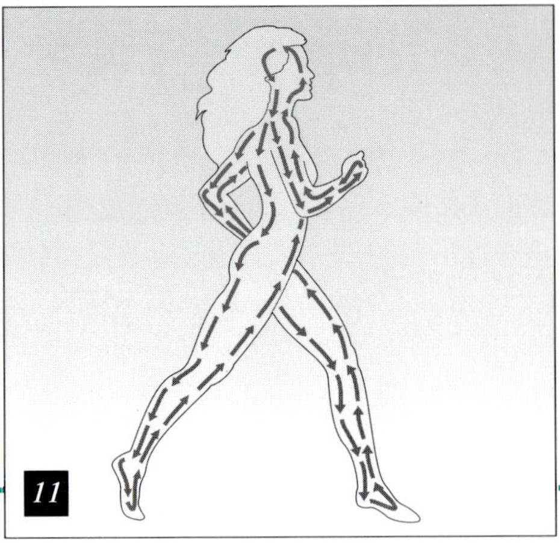
11

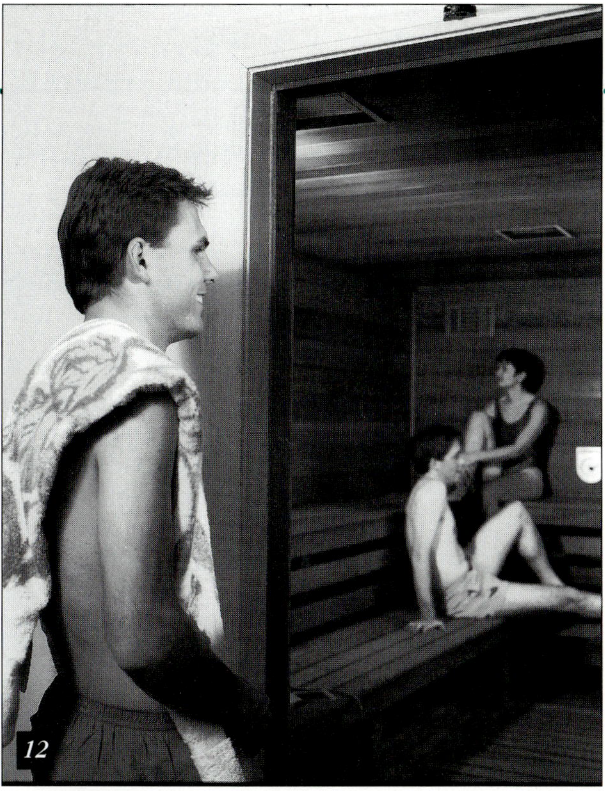

After running, the person sweats out the drug residuals in a sauna. Profuse sweating helps purify the system of these toxic substances.

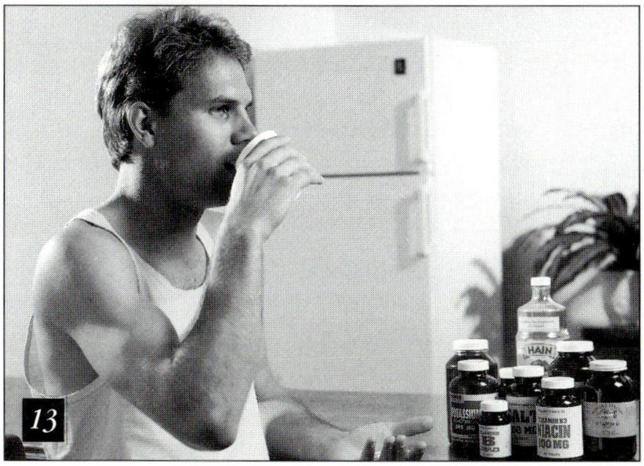

Nutrition in the form of certain vitamins and minerals is also an important part of the program.

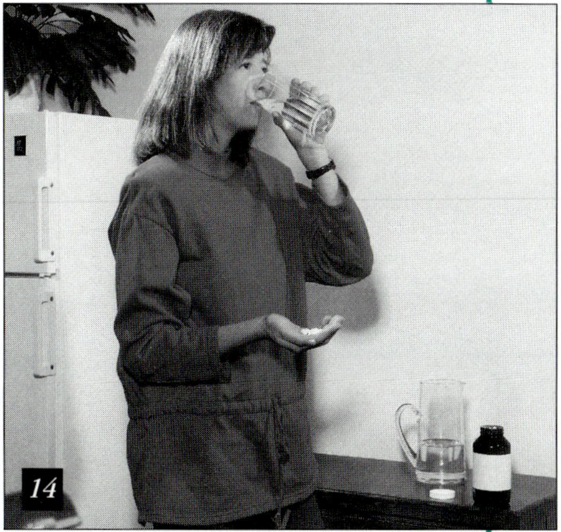

Niacin, one of the B complex vitamins, plays a vital role. It appears to break up and unleash drug and chemical deposits from body tissues and cells.

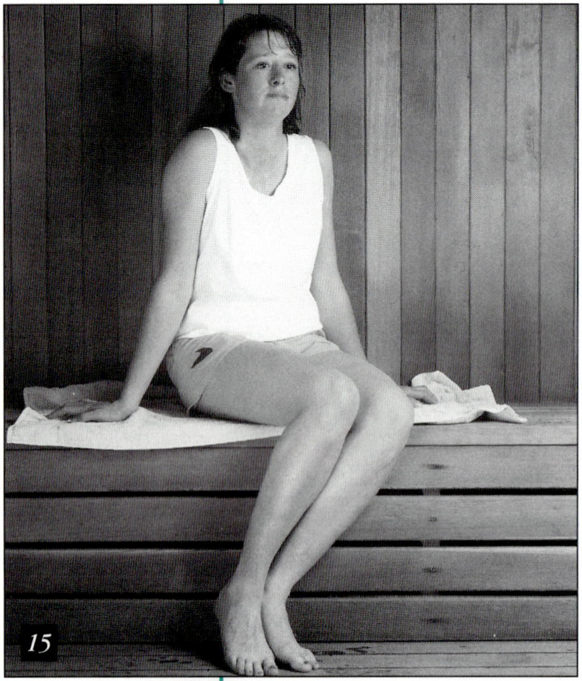

Niacin can produce some dramatic effects, such as a hot flush, as it interacts with deficiencies which already exist in cellular structure.

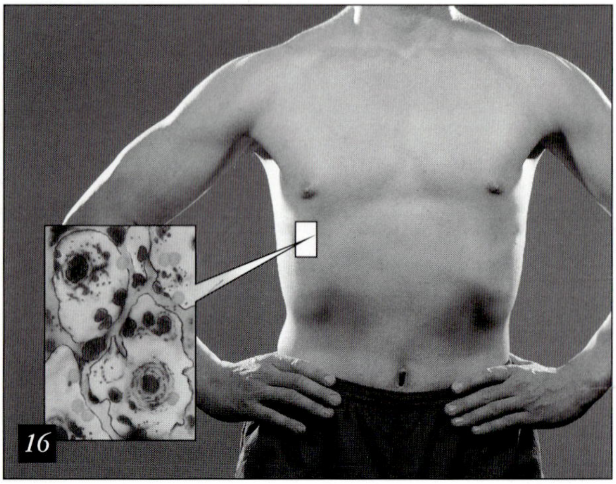

Because drug residues tend to "lock up" in fatty tissues . . .

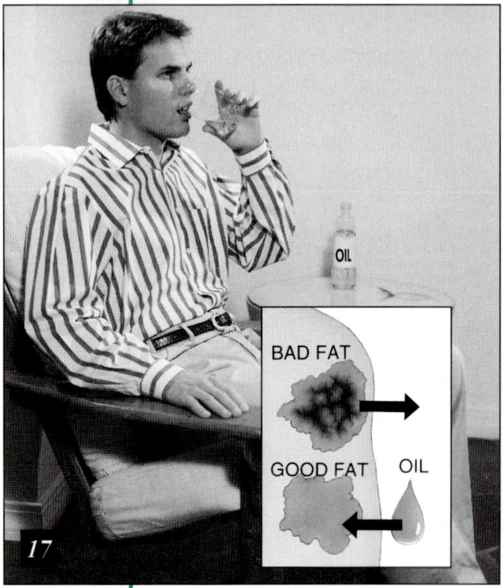

. . . some oil is taken every day to encourage bad, drug-laden fat to exchange with good oil.

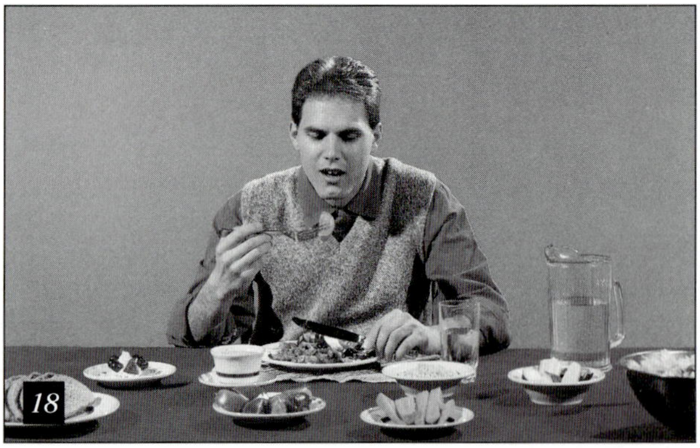

The person continues to eat his regular diet, ensuring he gets plenty of vegetables (which are not overcooked).

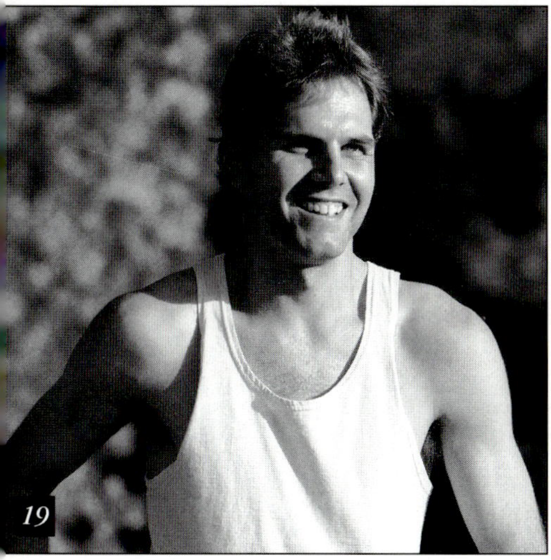

19

The regimen of running . .

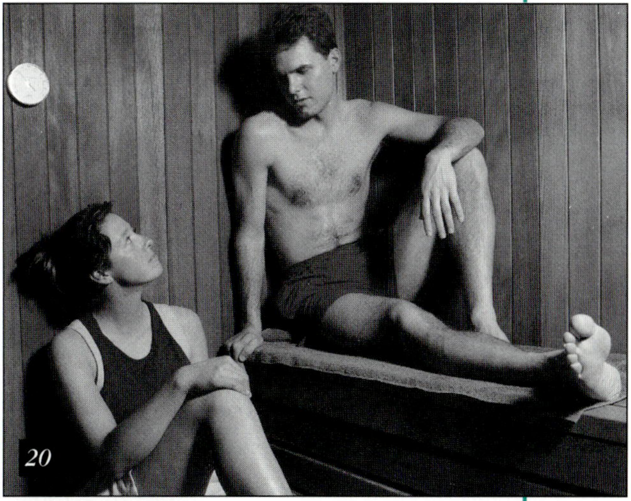

20

. . . sweating in a sauna, nutrition, and adequate rest is repeated daily . . .

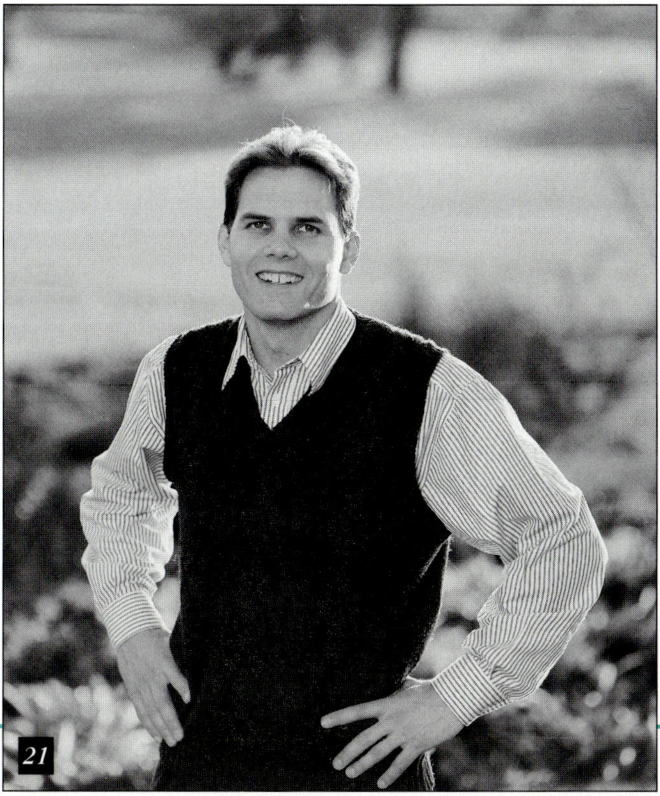

21

. . . until one no longer feels the effects of past drugs going into restimulation. The Purification program puts a person in a position where he can make real mental and spiritual gains with Scientology processing, because the effects of drugs on the mind and spirit are not constantly being put into restimulation.

The purpose of this program is very simply to clean out and purify one's system of all the accumulated impurities such as drugs, insecticides and pesticides, food preservatives, etc., which by their presence and restimulative effects could prevent or delay freeing the being spiritually through further Scientology processing. For someone who has taken LSD or angel dust this would include getting rid of any residual crystals from the body.

As the person goes through the Purification program, one should be able to see an improvement in his physical well-being as he rids the system of its accumulated impurities. The result of this program is a purified body, free from the impurities, drugs, etc., that had accumulated in it. We are not concerned with handling bodies with the Purification program, however. Our concern is freeing the individual up spiritually.

The Purification program is available under expert supervision in Scientology organizations and missions around the world. Also the book *Clear Body, Clear Mind: The Effective Purification Program* tells one exactly how this program is administered and describes all of its steps.

One should be able to get through the whole program in two weeks at five hours a day. Some will take more and some will take less.

With the Purification program we now have the means to get rapid recovery from the effects of the accumulation of the environmental chemical poisons as well as the medical drugs and street drugs which inhibit a person mentally and spiritually.

With the inclusion of vitamins, minerals and oils we are able to work toward restoring the biochemical balance of the body and make it possible for the body to reconstruct itself from the damage done by drugs and other biochemical substances.

The Drug Rundown

While the Purification program is a vital step in handling the effects of drugs, it is not a full handling in itself.

Complete freedom from drugs and their damaging consequences requires that a person also directly address the mental image pictures that are connected with having taken drugs. While the Purification program gets rid of drug residues that keep mental image pictures in constant restimulation, these pictures still exist. They can be restimulated by perceptions in the environment and affect the person adversely, below his awareness and out of his control, a factor that is both insidious and extremely detrimental.

The processing which directly deals with these pictures is called the Drug Rundown. It is delivered by highly trained practitioners in Scientology churches and missions.

A *rundown* is a series of steps designed to handle a specific aspect of a person's life or difficulties and which has a known end result. The result of the Drug Rundown is freedom from the harmful effects of drugs, alcohol and medicine and freedom from the need to take them.

A person's perceptions and recordings of the physical universe when on drugs are inaccurate, to say the least, as they are a combination of past events, imagination and the actual events which occurred at the time. A person can have pictures from past experiences tangled up with his present time perceptions. In essence, then, the pictures in his mind are scrambled to one degree or another. Thus his memory and his ability to think are both impaired.

The Drug Rundown handles several major aspects of past drug use. First, experiences the person had while taking drugs are directly addressed with precise procedures, which free up attention that became stuck on those experiences so they no longer affect him.

Normally, a person accurately records in his mind perceptions of the physical universe.

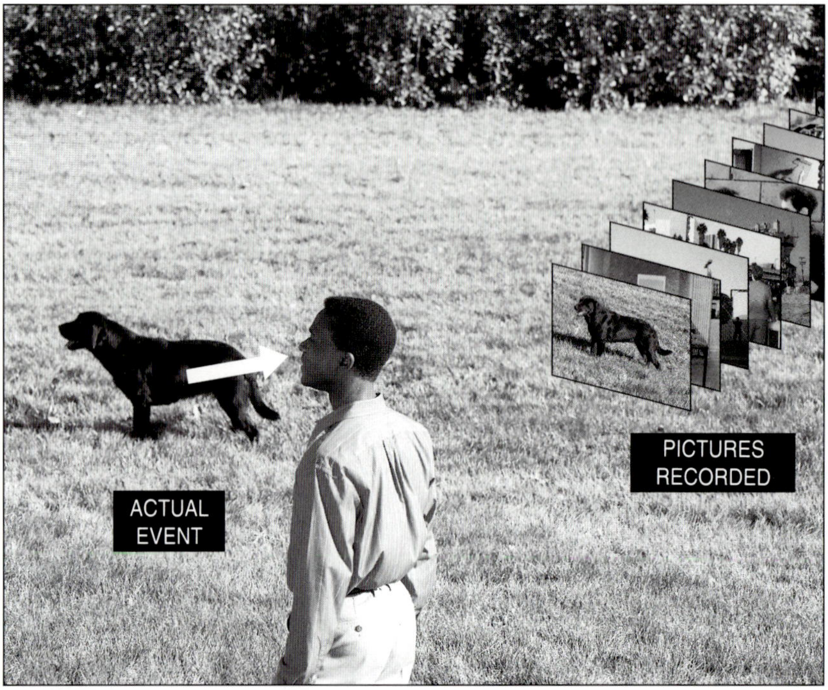

But drugs can tangle these recordings and badly distort what he perceives and, later, his recollection of what actually occurred.

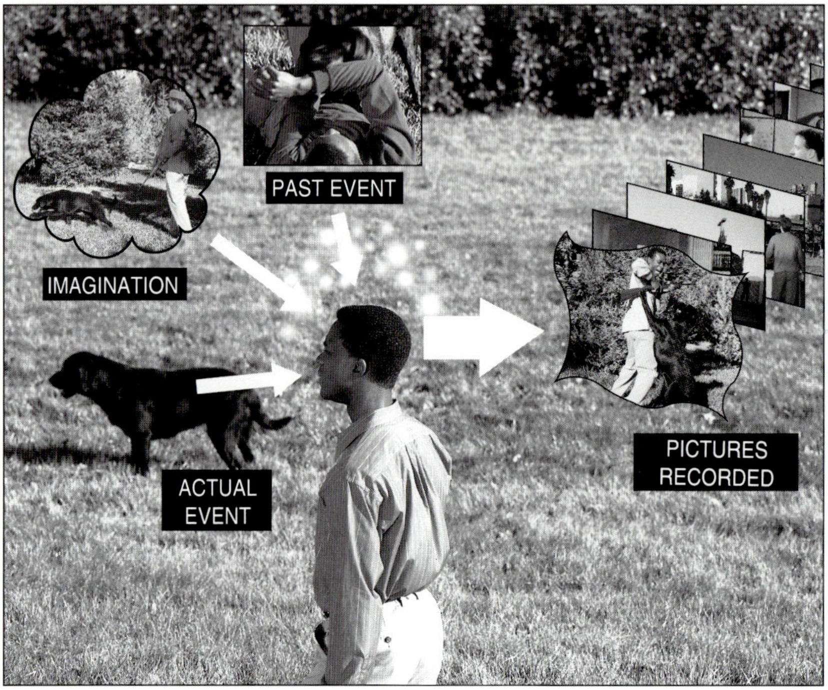

The more a person has had his attention freed from past incidents, the more able he is to deal with his life. He feels brighter, has increased perception, is better able to control himself and the things in his surroundings, and he becomes more able to rationally interact with others.

Another factor addressed by the Drug Rundown is that a person who has taken drugs also has a host of unpleasant physical, emotional and mental sensations connected with them. By discovering and examining the source of these, the harmful energy connected with them in the mind is released.

Finally, the processing gets right to the core of the matter and locates the basic reasons a person took drugs. A person originally turned to drugs for a *reason*—some physical suffering or hopelessness. The drug problem is thus essentially spiritual. The being was somehow suffering and drugs became a way to alleviate this.

The person looked upon drugs, alcohol or medicine as a cure for unwanted feelings or conditions—which could cover an almost infinite spectrum, and include anything from physical pains to anxiety to lack of confidence. One, therefore, has to find out what was actually wrong *before* drugs became his solution or "cure."

If this original reason is not addressed, the need or compulsion to take drugs or medicine or alcohol remains. Processing not only effectively deals with the effects of drugs, but enables the person to discover and eradicate the causes which led him to take them in the first place, thereby completely eliminating any desire to use or depend on them in the future.

The Drug Rundown, therefore, deals with and handles the unwanted feelings the person had both during *and* prior to the use of drugs, alcohol or medicine. The compulsion to still use drugs or alcohol is removed so that the person has no need to ever again turn to them.

By completing this processing, the person is at last free from any effects of drugs.

A full resolution of the mental and spiritual damage from past drug use requires *all* these steps.

A person can locate the source of any harmful mental effects of drugs, alcohol and medicine with Drug Rundown processing. The person can become free from those harmful mental effects and, as well, free from the need to take drugs ever again.

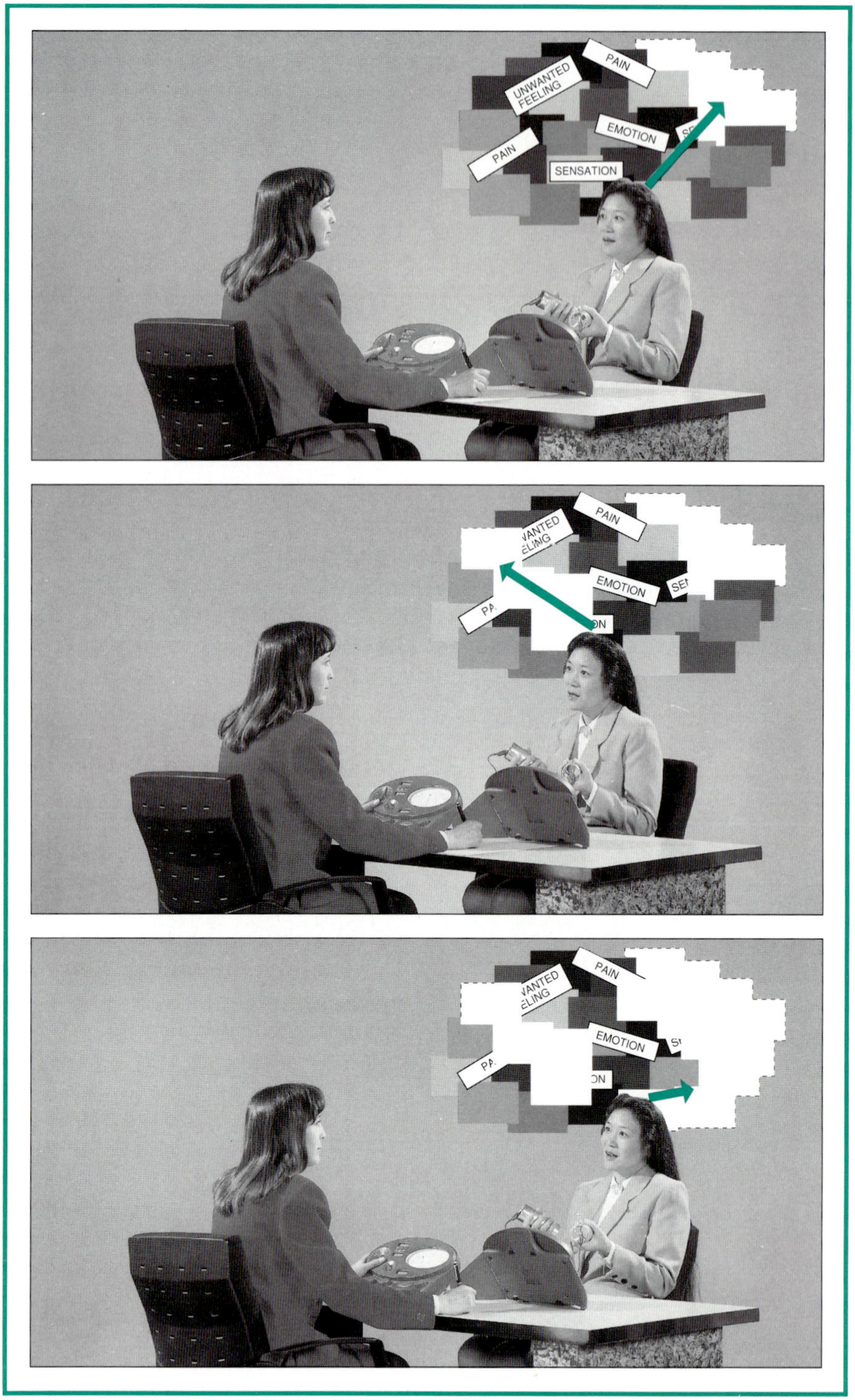

THE ROAD OUT

Only Scientology can fully handle the effects of drugs.

The means to get someone off drugs are now known—nutritional handling and Objective Processes which help the person get through any period of "drying out."

The next action, then, is the Purification program. This program is for any person who has taken drugs or anyone subjected to toxic substances of any kind.

And after a person has successfully finished the Purification program, processing on the Drug Rundown fully completes handling of the mental and spiritual effects of drugs.

Without workable methods to handle the effects of drugs, many people are doomed to live in chemical shackles. While drugs may appear to have short-term benefits, they only mask problems, they don't solve them.

Other drug rehabilitation approaches have failed mainly because of a lack of knowledge. They lack a true understanding of the mind, there is little or no understanding of man's spiritual nature, and the effects of drugs upon the mind and the being are unknown. The result is a materialistic ("man is an animal") approach which ignores these fundamental and crucial factors. All this adds up to proven unworkability.

Scientology, on the other hand, has a workable and extremely effective drug rehabilitation program because it addresses not only the correct problems, but the real sources of those problems.

Through understanding of the true nature of man, the methods to handle the biochemical, mental and spiritual factors of drugs do exist.

Scientology has the answers. ■

Practical Exercises

Here are exercises you can do to help increase your understanding of and ability to apply the data in this booklet.

1 Look around the place where you live or work and find examples of drugs or toxins. For instance, look at the labels of any products that may be in a medicine cabinet, or food labels, etc. Do this until you can easily recognize examples of drugs and toxins in your environment.

2 Look around your environment and note examples of the effects of drug use in society.

3 Obtain the ingredients for Cal-Mag and make a glass of it, following the directions in the booklet.

4 Find a friend or someone you know who has used drugs and process him on one of the Objective Processes given in this booklet until the person has good indicators and has had a cognition as a result of the process. Repeat this with other people you know until you feel confident in your ability to use these processes.

5 Educate someone on the subject of drugs using data from this booklet, with the end result that the person knows what drugs are and their effects, and the only effective solutions for them, as discovered in Scientology.

RESULTS FROM APPLICATION

Government-funded drug rehabilitation programs around the world continue to fail with a lamentable average success rate of 15 percent. This means that eighty-five out of one hundred addicts continue their habits—and is no success at all. But drug rehabilitation programs which use L. Ron Hubbard's technology almost reverse this failing ratio. An independent study in Spain, for instance, showed that 70 percent of graduates from a program based on Mr. Hubbard's work stayed off drugs. In Sweden, another independent study reported that 84 percent of graduates from a similar program were still drug-free two years after completion.

SCIENTOLOGY PROMOTES DRUG-FREE LIVING

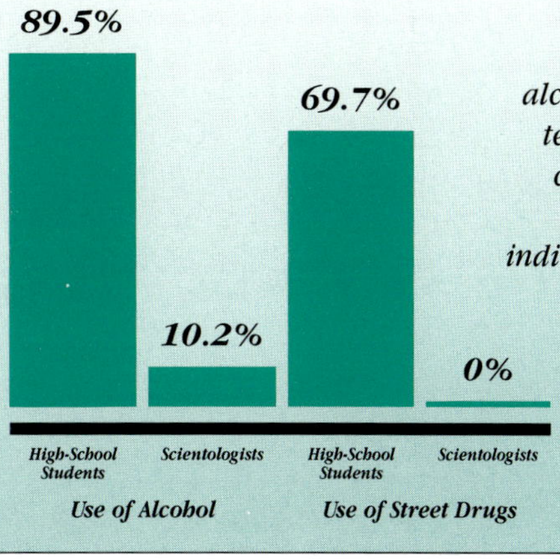

A comparison of drug and alcohol use by US teenagers and a cross section of Scientologists indicates the value of Scientology in solving the drug problem.

Mr. Hubbard's drug rehabilitation program is delivered in Scientology organizations throughout the world. If you run into any difficulty applying any of the procedures in this booklet, and require assistance, you may contact the nearest church or mission listed at the back of the booklet.

The effectiveness of using Mr. Hubbard's methods to salvage others from the devastating effects of drug use—and the sense of achievement gained from doing so—is reflected in the following pages:

After starting to use drugs at the age of thirteen, an American man finally admitted to himself nine years later that he was a drug addict. He decided to do something to get off cocaine and other drugs before they destroyed his life totally. Here is his story:

"I joined the US military because I thought the discipline would help me kick my habit and stay away from drugs, but as a gunner paratrooper, I ended up using as much cocaine as I had in civilian life. About a quarter of my division used drugs and we called ourselves the 'flying junkies.' So I left the military after three years because of drug use. I obviously needed something other than military life to help me handle my problem. I began to drift in and out of various drug programs over the next five years. However it wasn't until I used L. Ron Hubbard's technology that I was able to live a drug-free life. Since that time, I have been helping others kick their addictions to everything from heroin to alcohol, using the program."

The Purification program is the only truly effective program of its kind in the world, as a medical doctor in Amsterdam, Holland agrees. After examining drug users before, during and after the Purification program, he said:

"In my opinion, the Purification program which was developed by L. Ron Hubbard is the only one which has

proved to be effective in practice. I speak from experience because I have had contact with addicts before they started the detoxification step of the Purification program. By doing the preparatory steps at the beginning of the program, the person has already changed so much that I sometimes think I have made a mistake and am not sitting opposite a former heroin addict."

Reflections of a father about his son, Robert, over a four-year span:

"Four years ago, Robert came home from Marine training, very quiet and withdrawn, with no interest in work or play; no normal drive to find his way in the world. He seemed to become worse by the week, very listless and depressed; being very naive, I never thought drugs to be the problem.

"After many visits to doctors and clinics, the doctors settled on prescribing the mind-bending drug, Ritalin, to 'improve his way of thinking.' This drug, being federally controlled, was supposed to help him in getting started on a 'normal way of thinking' and doing things other 'normal' people do.

"Robert became addicted to this drug to the extent of hundreds of pills each week. Even though the drug was supposedly controlled, unscrupulous doctors prescribed the medication. He became a legal dope addict. In my state of mind, I called up these doctors and threatened legal action, but Robert would just find another doctor who was anxious to make a fast dollar and get more medication.

"He became so hard to live with and so mean that he would steal from us and lie to and threaten his mother. I finally had him arrested for grand theft just to get him out of the house and in the hope of shocking him into reality. The judge let him out on probation, and he went on taking Ritalin.

"We were at a breaking point and were considering having him sent to prison before he hurt himself or I hurt him (God forbid).

"I was watching television one morning and saw two young men speaking about drug problems and insisting that they could help if one would just call, so I did. Then I talked to my son and we set up a meeting. So Robert went off to a center in Los Angeles that uses Mr. Hubbard's technology. They began to work with him on a twenty-four-hour basis to help him get off drugs.

"Robert began to change for the better—and oh, what a change. No more drugs. He came home on weekends, and was calm and collected and began to talk intelligently and act sanely.

"Four months have passed, and Robert has improved by the week, no longer harassing his mother, no more asking for the impossible or 'twisting' things to suit his way.

"He has really beat the drug and is well on his way to doing something worthwhile.

"Our friends and others now ask how we came to have a son who is so considerate, calm and intelligent-speaking. I just smile and reply that he

works with a group of people in Los Angeles that help young people get started on the road of life.

"Good luck, Robert,

from your Dad.

"And thanks to all his friends there, at the center."

The joy of creating was restored to a musician when she was able to shed the effects of drugs.

"As a musician, one of the most important abilities is to be highly aware of what the other players are doing and thinking. While on the Purification program I handled the effects of a lot of marijuana and also medical anesthetics.

"One day my awareness sort of popped up to a completely new level—colors, sounds . . . all my perceptions were wider and richer. I was pretty excited about this; however, the best was yet to come. That night I went to rehearsal and right from the start I could tell that something was different and better. As a group we were what we call "in the pocket" all night—that incredible state where you are closely and intensely aware of what each person is doing and where they're going. All your attention is off yourself and the mechanics of playing and totally on the creation of the music!

"It was effortless and stable. The audience **and** *the band members were all amazed at the difference.*

"That feeling is priceless."

Years of addiction to heroin had brought a married couple to the brink of death with no road out. Fortunately the husband's sister introduced them to Mr. Hubbard's discoveries concerning drugs and they were able to restore their health and zest for life.

"When my husband and I started Mr. Hubbard's drug rehabilitation program we were both heroin addicts and used other drugs too. My husband had been told by three doctors that he didn't have long to live. He was having repeated seizures; his heart and breathing even stopped at three different times and I was barely able to save him. We were at our wits' end when my husband's sister told us about Mr. Hubbard's drug rehabilitation technology.

"We found a center that delivered the program and went through withdrawal—which was surprisingly easy. We were amazed at how fast and efficiently it worked, especially considering the amount of drugs we had used.

"Then we went onto the Purification program. The sauna was very tough but it helped to sweat all the old drugs out of our bodies. When my husband was done he said he felt as though a fog had just lifted from his head. I felt like a teenager again, all young and vibrant. As for the rest of the program, it helped to get the cravings out of my head and got me into present time so that I wasn't dwelling on the past.

"The program gave me a new outlook on life. I have no more cravings for drugs and I have my husband back in full force. He seems to have no problems with anything. He is as healthy as anyone that has never done drugs before.

"I want to thank the people of the center for giving us our lives back and letting us live happily, healthily and drug-free.

"We have decided to stay on at the center to help others achieve drug-free lives and try to make this whole planet drug-free. I feel like I could accomplish anything. I feel young again, not under the weight of those drugs that held me down so long."

A mother in Milan, Italy, was in despair as she watched her son deteriorate under the devastating effects of drugs. Her despair turned to hope and then happiness as her son was restored to her through Mr. Hubbard's drug rehabilitation technology.

"The hope that my son could be free of drugs was with me for many years. But day after day I felt him going away from me. I saw the moment of his rehabilitation far, far away.

"Then my son enrolled in a drug rehabilitation center using Mr. Hubbard's technology. I have to confess that I didn't believe it would work. He was at the center for about eight months, but I feared that once back home he would start taking drugs again, as we had had similar experiences in the past. But I told myself to have faith and courage once more.

"It's been four years now that my son has been completely fine. He never reverted to drugs, has a good job and I see him very self-confident in things he does."

Existence was a downhill slide toward total disaster for one Englishman until a friend helped him stop, turn around and climb back up to a life worth living.

"Before I came across Mr. Hubbard's drug rehabilitation program, I had been using drugs for sixteen years. I started out smoking marijuana and soon progressed to amphetamines, LSD and sleeping pills. This carried on for about ten years before I got involved in the 'fashionable' abuse of cocaine. I really thought that I was in touch with what life was about. But that was just the effect of my mind and body which, I now know, were thoroughly polluted with the drugs (poisons) I'd been taking. All the time this was going on, I couldn't hold down any responsible jobs or take any responsibility for the normal business of everyday life.

"Crime became the other side of my life. As my need for more drugs grew, so did the seriousness of the crimes I committed. I became very withdrawn into myself and found it hard to have normal conversations about anything. My powers of self-control were totally shot away and after a particular criminal incident, I once again found myself in jail. Because my morale was very low, heroin was a comfortable form of escape from the reality of what was happening to my life. After three months in jail I was released back into society to continue where I had left off. But unfortunately, for myself and society, I was now addicted to heroin.

"All my hopes and ambitions had blown away and now I was on the inevitable downward slope. Crime once again became an everyday affair. But I had no control whatsoever and before I realized what I was doing, I had gotten myself into more serious trouble than ever.

"Finally, at the urging of my family, I started the long battle to overcome my addictions. I suffered numerous uncomfortable and unsuccessful detoxifications in various clinics which cost me in excess of $25,000. But within a very short time of each detoxification, I was back on heroin again. I couldn't understand why, after each time I returned to society with positive intentions, I wound up back in the frame of mind that I couldn't handle life without heroin.

"Fortunately, I found somebody who knew about the incredible success of Mr. Hubbard's drug rehabilitation techniques. I started the program and after only a very short time, I had put control into my life—probably for the first time.

"Since finishing the program I know that I have a future and that I can live the rest of my life as the rest of my life, not just 'day by day.'

"If you are looking for a way out, here it is. I know."

There are many who never succumb to the pressures and enticements toward drug abuse all too common in today's society. But even these people are unlikely to escape the effects of the many harmful substances that pervade the modern world—pesticides, industrial wastes, air pollution, food preservatives and additives; the list goes on. Mr. Hubbard's Purification program offers an answer to the adverse spiritual effects of this chemical assault. For this reason, the Purification program has found wide appeal not only with those who have been subjected to the ravages of street drugs, but to those who have led relatively drug-free lives. The story that follows exemplifies this fact.

"Before doing the Purification program I was not what you would call a 'druggie' at all. I'd had some drinks and been given medical drugs a few times, but that was all. I didn't think that these would have had much effect on me. Nonetheless, when I heard about the Purification program I was interested right away. I thought that all the chemicals I'd taken in over the years, in packaged foods, bad city air, tap water and so on might be having some effect on me. Well, I was right!

"After doing the program the change in me was incredible. I used to get headaches all the time. I thought it was just something I would have to live with. After the Purification program they went away and have never come back.

"But more importantly, I felt completely pure and much more in present time. Very fresh and alert and 'there.' It made a big difference."

About L. Ron Hubbard

No more fitting statement typifies the life of L. Ron Hubbard than his simple declaration: "I like to help others and count it as my greatest pleasure in life to see a person free himself from the shadows which darken his days." Behind these pivotal words stands a lifetime of service to mankind and a legacy of wisdom that enables anyone to attain long-cherished dreams of happiness and spiritual freedom.

Born in Tilden, Nebraska on March 13, 1911, his road of discovery and dedication to his fellows began at an early age. "I wanted other people to be happy, and could not understand why they weren't," he wrote of his youth; and therein lay the sentiments that would long guide his steps. By the age of nineteen, he had traveled more than a quarter of a million miles, examining the cultures of Java, Japan, India and the Philippines.

Returning to the United States in 1929, Ron resumed his formal education and studied mathematics, engineering and the then new field of nuclear physics—all providing vital tools for continued research. To finance that research, Ron embarked upon a literary career in the early 1930s, and soon became one of the most widely read authors of popular fiction. Yet never losing sight of his primary goal, he continued his mainline research through extensive travel and expeditions.

With the advent of World War II, he entered the United States Navy as a lieutenant (junior grade) and served as commander of antisubmarine corvettes. Left partially blind and lame from injuries sustained during combat, he was diagnosed as permanently disabled by 1945. Through application of his theories on the mind, however, he was not only able to help fellow servicemen, but also to regain his own health.

After five more years of intensive research, Ron's discoveries were presented to the world in *Dianetics: The Modern Science of Mental Health.* The first popular handbook on the human mind expressly written for the man in the street, *Dianetics* ushered in a new era of hope for mankind and a new phase of life for its author. He did, however, not cease his research, and as breakthrough after breakthrough was carefully codified through late 1951, the applied religious philosophy of Scientology was born.

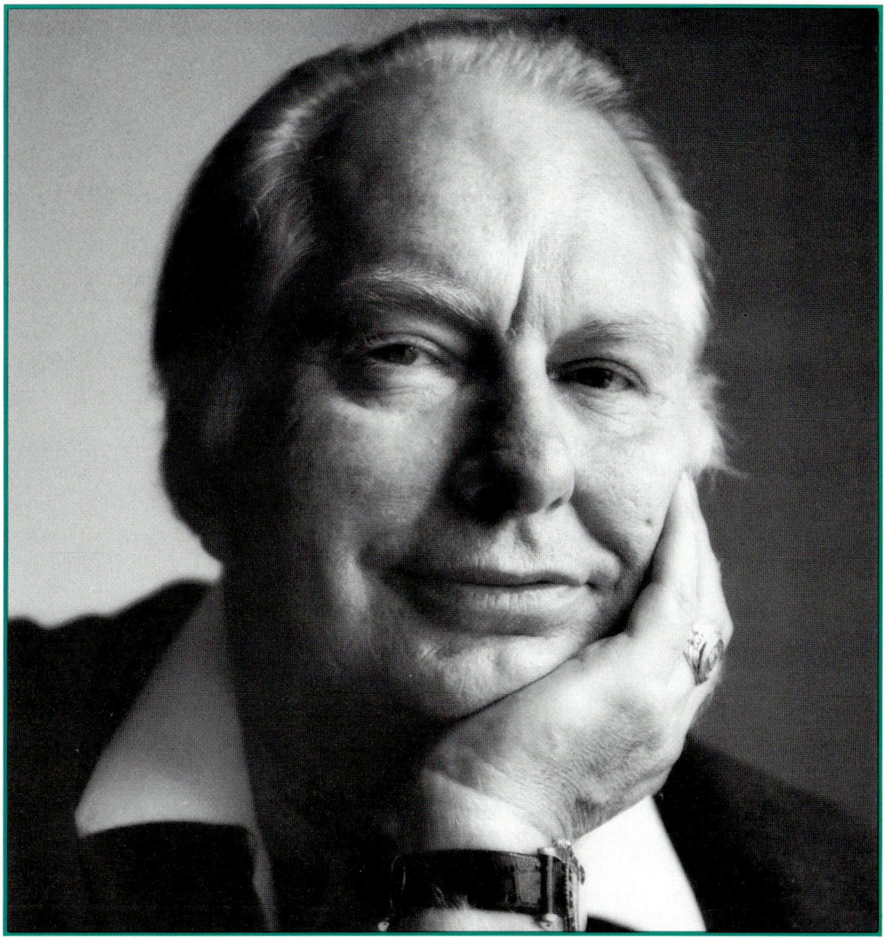

Because Scientology explains the whole of life, there is no aspect of man's existence that L. Ron Hubbard's subsequent work did not address. Residing variously in the United States and England, his continued research brought forth solutions to such social ills as declining educational standards and pandemic drug abuse.

All told, L. Ron Hubbard's works on Scientology and Dianetics total forty million words of recorded lectures, books and writings. Together, these constitute the legacy of a lifetime that ended on January 24, 1986. Yet the passing of L. Ron Hubbard in no way constituted an end; for with a hundred million of his books in circulation and millions of people daily applying his technologies for betterment, it can truly be said the world still has no greater friend. ■

Glossary

acknowledge: give (someone) an acknowledgment. *See also* **acknowledgment** in this glossary.

acknowledgment: something said or done to inform another that his statement or action has been noted, understood and received.

auditing: same as *processing. See* **processing** in this glossary.

auditor: someone who is trained and qualified to apply Scientology processing to individuals for their benefit. The term comes from the Latin *audire,* "to listen." *See also* **processing** in this glossary.

cognition: a new realization about life. It is a "What do you know, I . . ." statement; something a person suddenly understands or feels.

Drug Rundown: a series of processes that address the mental image pictures connected with having taken drugs. The result of the Drug Rundown is freedom from the harmful effects of drugs, alcohol and medicine, and freedom from the need to take them.

havingness: the feeling that one owns or possesses; it can also be described as the concept of being able to reach or not being prevented from reaching.

indicator: a condition or circumstance arising during a process which indicates (points out or shows) whether the process is going well or badly. For example, the person receiving the processing looking brighter or looking more cheerful would be good indicators. *See also* **process** in this glossary.

mental image pictures: three-dimensional color pictures with sound and smell and all other perceptions, plus the conclusions or speculations of the individual. They are mental copies of one's perceptions sometime in the past, although in cases of unconsciousness or lessened consciousness they exist *below* the individual's awareness.

Objective Process: a type of process which helps a person direct his attention off himself and onto his environment and the people and things in it. *Objective* refers to outward things, not the thoughts or feelings of the individual. *Objective Processes* deal with the real and observable. They call for the person to spot or find something exterior to himself. *See also* **process** in this glossary.

present time: the time which is now and becomes the past as rapidly as it is observed. It is a term loosely applied to the environment existing in now.

process: an exact series of directions or sequence of actions taken to accomplish a desired result.

processing: a special form of personal counseling, unique in Scientology, which helps an individual look at his own existence and improves his ability to confront what he is and where he is. Processing is a precise, thoroughly codified activity with exact procedures.

Purification Rundown: a program of exercise, sauna sweat-out, nutrition and properly ordered personal schedule. It cleans out and purifies one's system of all the accumulated impurities such as drugs, insecticides and pesticides, food preservatives, etc., which by their presence and restimulative effects could prevent or delay freeing the being spiritually through Scientology processing.

reality: that which appears to be. Reality is fundamentally agreement; the degree of agreement reached by people. What we agree to be real is real.

restimulation: the reactivation of a memory of a past unpleasant experience due to similar circumstances in the present approximating circumstances of the past.

rundown: a series of steps designed to handle a specific aspect of a person's life or difficulties and which has a known end result.

Scientology: an applied religious philosophy developed by L. Ron Hubbard. It is the study and handling of the spirit in relationship to itself, universes and other life. The word *Scientology* comes from the Latin *scio,* which means "know" and the Greek word *logos,* meaning "the word or outward form by which the inward thought is expressed and made known." Thus, Scientology means knowing about knowing.

somatic: a word used in Scientology to designate any body sensation, illness, pain or discomfort. *Soma* means "body" in Greek.

thetan: the person himself—not his body or his name, the physical universe, his mind or anything else—it is that which is aware of being aware; the identity which *is* the individual. The term *thetan* was coined to eliminate any possible confusion with older, invalid concepts. It comes from the Greek letter *theta* which the Greeks used to represent *thought* or perhaps *spirit,* to which an *n* is added to make a noun in the modern style used to create words in engineering.

time track: the accumulated record of all one's mental image pictures. *See also* **mental image pictures** in this glossary.

TR: abbreviation for *T*raining *R*outine. *See* **Training Routines** in this glossary.

Training Routines: training drills that enable a person to improve his level of communication skill. By doing these drills any person's ability to communicate with others can be vastly improved.

HURCHES OF SCIENTOLOGY

ESTERN UNITED ATES

rch of Scientology of Arizona
1 W. University Dr.
a, Arizona 85201

rch of Scientology of the Valley
9 West Magnolia Boulevard
bank, California 91506

rch of Scientology of
s Angeles
) Sunset Boulevard
Angeles, California 90027

rch of Scientology of
lountain View
3 Old Middlefield Way
ntain View, California 96043

rch of Scientology of
asadena
E. Colorado Boulevard
dena, California 91101

rch of Scientology of
cramento
15th Street
amento, California 95814

rch of Scientology of
n Diego
"C" Street, Suite 200
Diego, California 92101

rch of Scientology of
n Francisco
IcAllister Street
Francisco, California 94102

rch of Scientology of
evens Creek
. Rosemary
Jose, California 95112

rch of Scientology of
nta Barbara
State Street
a Barbara, California 93101

rch of Scientology of
range County
Irvine Boulevard
in, California 92680

rch of Scientology of Colorado
S. Navajo Street
ver, Colorado 80223

Church of Scientology of Hawaii
1146 Bethel Street
Honolulu, Hawaii 96813

Church of Scientology of Minnesota
Twin Cities
1011 Nicollet Mall
Minneapolis, Minnesota 55403

Church of Scientology of Kansas City
3619 Broadway
Kansas City, Missouri 64111

Church of Scientology of Missouri
9510 Page Boulevard
St. Louis, Missouri 63132

Church of Scientology of Nevada
846 E. Sahara Avenue
Las Vegas, Nevada 89104

Church of Scientology of New Mexico
8106 Menaul Boulevard N.E.
Albuquerque, New Mexico 87110

Church of Scientology of Portland
323 S.W. Washington
Portland, Oregon 97204

Church of Scientology of Texas
2200 Guadalupe
Austin, Texas 78705

Church of Scientology of Utah
1931 S. 1100 East
Salt Lake City, Utah 84106

Church of Scientology of Washington State
2226 3rd Avenue
Seattle, Washington 98121

EASTERN UNITED STATES

Church of Scientology of Connecticut
909 Whalley Avenue
New Haven, Connecticut 06515

Church of Scientology of Florida
120 Giralda Avenue
Coral Gables, Florida 33134

Church of Scientology of Orlando
1830 East Colonial Drive
Orlando, Florida 32803

Church of Scientology of Tampa
3617 Henderson Boulevard
Tampa, Florida 33609

Church of Scientology of Georgia
2632 Piedmont Road, N.E.
Atlanta, Georgia 30324

Church of Scientology of Illinois
3011 N. Lincoln Avenue
Chicago, Illinois 60657

Church of Scientology of Boston
448 Beacon Street
Boston, Massachusetts 02115

Church of Scientology of Ann Arbor
2355 West Stadium Boulevard
Ann Arbor, Michigan 48103

Church of Scientology of Michigan
321 Williams Street
Royal Oak, Michigan 48067

Church of Scientology of Buffalo
47 West Huron Street
Buffalo, New York 14202

Church of Scientology of Long Island
99 Railroad Station Plaza
Hicksville, New York 11801

Church of Scientology of New York
227 West 46th Street
New York City, New York 10036

Church of Scientology of Cincinnati
215 West 4th Street, 5th Floor
Cincinnati, Ohio 45202

Church of Scientology of Ohio
30 North High Street
Columbus, Ohio 43215

Church of Scientology of Pennsylvania
1315 Race Street
Philadelphia, Pennsylvania 19107

Founding Church of Scientology of Washington, DC
2125 "S" Street N.W.
Washington, DC 20008

PUERTO RICO

Church of Scientology of Puerto Rico
272 JT Piniero Avenue
Hyde Park, Hato Rey
Puerto Rico 00918

UNITED KINGDOM

Church of Scientology of Birmingham
Albert House, 3rd Floor
24 Albert Street
Birmingham
England B4 7UD

Church of Scientology of Brighton
5 St. Georges Place
London Road
Brighton, Sussex
England BN1 4GA

Church of Scientology Saint Hill Foundation
Saint Hill Manor
East Grinstead, West Sussex
England RH19 4JY

Church of Scientology of London
68 Tottenham Court Road
London
England W1P 0BB

Church of Scientology of Manchester
258 Deansgate
Manchester
England M3 4BG

Church of Scientology of Plymouth
41 Ebrington Street
Plymouth, Devon
England PL4 9AA

Church of Scientology of Sunderland
51 Fawcett Street
Sunderland, Tyne and Wear
England SR1 1RS

Hubbard Academy of Personal Independence
20 Southbridge
Edinburgh
Scotland EH1 1LL

Europe

Austria

Church of Scientology of Austria
Schottenfeldgasse 13/15
1070 Wien

Belgium

Church of Scientology of Belgium
61, rue du Prince Royal
1050 Bruxelles

Denmark

Church of Scientology of Jylland
Guldsmedegade 17, 2
8000 Aarhus C

Church of Scientology of Copenhagen
Store Kongensgade 55
1264 Copenhagen K

Church of Scientology of Denmark
Gammel Kongevej 3–5, 1
1610 Copenhagen V

France

Church of Scientology of Angers
10–12, rue Max Richard
49100 Angers

Church of Scientology of Clermont-Ferrand
1, rue Ballainvilliers
63000 Clermont-Ferrand

Church of Scientology of Lyon
3, place des Capucins
69001 Lyon

Church of Scientology of Paris
65, rue de Dunkerque
75009 Paris

Church of Scientology of Saint-Étienne
24, rue Marengo
42000 Saint-Étienne

Germany

Church of Scientology of Berlin
Sponholzstraße 51–52
12159 Berlin

Church of Scientology of Düsseldorf
Friedrichstraße 28
40217 Düsseldorf

Church of Scientology of Frankfurt
Darmstädter Landstraße 213
60598 Frankfurt

Church of Scientology of Hamburg
Steindamm 63
20099 Hamburg

Church of Scientology of Hanover
Hubertusstraße 2
30163 Hannover

Church of Scientology of Munich
Beichstraße 12
80802 München

Church of Scientology of Stuttgart
Urbanstraße 70
70182 Stuttgart

Israel

Dianetics and Scientology College of Israel
42 Gorden Street, 2nd Floor
Tel Aviv 66023

Italy

Church of Scientology of Brescia
Via Fratelli Bronzetti, 20
25125 Brescia

Church of Scientology of Catania
Via Garibaldi, 9
95121 Catania

Church of Scientology of Milan
Via Abetone, 10
20137 Milano

Church of Scientology of Monza
Via Cavour, 5
20052 Monza

Church of Scientology of Novara
Corso Cavallotti, 7
28100 Novara

Church of Scientology of Nuoro
Via Lamarmora, 115
08100 Nuoro

Church of Scientology of Padua
Via Mameli, 1/5
35131 Padova

Church of Scientology of Pordenone
Via Montereale, 10/C
33170 Pordenone

Church of Scientology of Rome
Via della Pineta Sacchetti, 201
00185 Roma

Church of Scientology of Turin
Via Bersezio, 7
10152 Torino

Church of Scientology of Verona
Via Vicolo Chiodo, 4/A
37121 Verona

Netherlands

Church of Scientology of Amsterdam
Nieuwe Zijds Voorburgwal 271
1012 RL Amsterdam

Norway

Church of Scientology of Norway
Storgata 9
0155 Oslo 1

Portugal

Church of Scientology of Portugal
Rua Actor Taborda 39–5°
1000 Lisboa

Russia

Hubbard Humanitarian Center
103064 Moscow
Homutovskiy Tupik 7, Russia

Spain

Dianetics Civil Association of Barcelona
C/ Pau Clarís 85, Principal dcha.
08010 Barcelona

Dianetics Civil Association of Madrid
C/ Montera 20, 1° dcha.
28013 Madrid

Sweden

Church of Scientology of Göteborg
Odinsgatan 8, 2 tr.
411 03 Göteborg

Church of Scientology of Malmö
Lantmannagatan 62 C
214 48 Malmö

Church of Scientology of Stockholm
St. Eriksgatan 56
112 34 Stockholm

Switzerland

Church of Scientology of Basel
Herrengrabenweg 56
4054 Basel

Church of Scientology of Bern
Dammweg 29
Postfach 352
3000 Bern 11

Church of Scientology of Geneva
Route de Saint-Julien 7–9 C.P. 823
1227 Carouge, Genève

Church of Scientology of Lausanne
10, rue de la Madeleine
1003 Lausanne

Church of Scientology of Zurich
Badenerstrasse 141
8004 Zurich

Africa

Church of Scientology of Cape Town
St. Georges Centre, 2nd Floor
13 Hout Street
Cape Town 8001
Republic of South Africa

Church of Scientology of Durban
57 College Lane
Durban 4001
Republic of South Africa

Church of Scientology of Johannesburg
Security Building, 2nd Floor
95 Commissioner Street
Johannesburg 2001
Republic of South Africa

Church of Scientology of Johannesburg North
1st Floor Bordeaux Centre
Gordon and Jan Smuts Ave.
Bordeaux, Randburg 2125
Republic of South Africa

Church of Scientology of Port Elizabeth
2 St. Christopher Place
27 Westbourne Road Central
Port Elizabeth 6001
Republic of South Africa

rch of Scientology of Pretoria
Ancore Building
e & Esselen Streets
oria 0002
ublic of South Africa

rch of Scientology of Bulawayo
hampton House, Suite 202
n Street and 9th Avenue
wayo
babwe

rch of Scientology of Harare
Box 3524
ivingston Road
re
babwe

STRALIA, W ZEALAND D OCEANIA

stralia

rch of Scientology of Adelaide
28 Waymouth Street
aide, South Australia 5000

rch of Scientology of Brisbane
Edward Street
bane, Queensland 4000

rch of Scientology of
ustralian Capital Territory
Bunda Street, Suite 16
: Canberra, A.C.T. 2601

rch of Scientology of
elbourne
4 Russell Street
bourne, Victoria 3000

rch of Scientology of Perth
1 King Street
n, Western Australia 6000

rch of Scientology of Sydney
Castlereagh Street
ey, New South Wales 2000

an

ntology Tokyo
1 Higashi Gotanda
agawa-ku
o, Japan 141

v Zealand

rch of Scientology
ew Zealand
orne Street
land 1

LATIN AMERICA

Colombia

Dianetics Cultural Center
Calle 95 No. 19-A-28
Barrio Chico, Bogotá

Mexico

Dianetics Cultural Organization, A.C.
Pedro Moreno 1078 Int 3
Sector Juárez,
Guadalajara, Jalisco

Dianetics Cultural Association, A.C.
Carrillo Puerto 54 Bis
Colonia Coyoacán
C.P. 04000, Mexico, D.F.

Latin American Cultural Center, A.C.
Durango 105
Colonia Roma
C.P. 03100, Mexico, D.F.

Institute of Applied Philosophy, A.C.
Juan de Dios Arias 83
Colonia Vista Alegre
Mexico, D.F.

Dianetics Technological Institute, A.C.
Avenida Juan Escutia 29
Colonia Condesa
Delegación Cuauhtemoc
C.P. 06140, Mexico, D.F.

Dianetics Development Organization, A.C.
Heriberto Frías 420
Colonia Narvarte
C.P. 03020, Mexico, D.F.

Dianetics Cultural Organization, A.C.
Nicolás San Juan 1734
Colonia del Valle
C.P. 03100, Mexico, D.F.

Venezuela

Dianetics Cultural Organization, A.C.
Avenida Principal de las Palmas,
Cruce Con Calle Carúpano
Quinta Suha, Las Palmas
Caracas

Dianetics Cultural Association, A.C.
Avenida 101, 150-23
Urbanización La Alegría
Apartado Postal 833
Valencia

CANADA

Church of Scientology of Edmonton
10187 112th Street
Edmonton, Alberta
Canada T5K 1M1

Church of Scientology of Kitchener
104 King Street West
Kitchener, Ontario
Canada N2G 2K6

Church of Scientology of Montreal
4489 Papineau Street
Montréal, Québec
Canada H2H 1T7

Church of Scientology of Ottawa
150 Rideau Street, 2nd Floor
Ottawa, Ontario
Canada K1N 5X6

Church of Scientology of Quebec
350 Bd Chareste Est
Québec, Québec
Canada G1K 3H5

Church of Scientology of Toronto
696 Yonge Street, 2nd Floor
Toronto, Ontario
Canada M4Y 2A7

Church of Scientology of Vancouver
401 West Hasting Street
Vancouver, British Columbia
Canada V6B 1L5

Church of Scientology of Winnipeg
388 Donald Street, Suite 125
Winnipeg, Manitoba
Canada R3B 2J4

CELEBRITY CENTRES

Church of Scientology
Celebrity Centre International
5930 Franklin Avenue
Hollywood, California 90028

Church of Scientology
Celebrity Centre Dallas
10500 Steppington Drive, Suite 100
Dallas, Texas 75230

Church of Scientology
Celebrity Centre Las Vegas
1100 South 10th Street
Las Vegas, Nevada 89104

Church of Scientology
Celebrity Centre Nashville
38 Music Square West
Nashville, Tennessee 37203

Church of Scientology
Celebrity Centre New York
65 East 82nd Street
New York City, New York 10036

Church of Scientology
Celebrity Centre Portland
709 Southwest Salmon Street
Portland, Oregon 97205

Church of Scientology
Celebrity Centre Washington, DC
4214 16th Street N.W.
Washington, DC 20011

Church of Scientology
Celebrity Centre London
27 Westbourne Grove
London W2, England

Church of Scientology
Celebrity Centre Vienna
Senefeldergasse 11/5
1100 Wien, Austria

Church of Scientology
Celebrity Centre Paris
69, rue Legendre
75017 Paris, France

Church of Scientology
Celebrity Centre Düsseldorf
Grupellostraße 28
40210 Düsseldorf, Germany

Church of Scientology
Celebrity Centre Hamburg
Eppendorfer Landstraße 35
20249 Hamburg, Germany

Church of Scientology
Celebrity Centre Munich
Landshuter Allee 42
80637 München, Germany

Scientology Missions

International Office

Scientology Missions International
6331 Hollywood Boulevard,
Suite 501
Los Angeles, California 90028

- ▲ Scientology Missions International Expansion Office
  210 South Fort Harrison Avenue
  Clearwater, Florida 34616

Western United States

- ▲ Scientology Missions International
  Western United States Office
  1307 N. New Hampshire,
  Suite 101
  Los Angeles, California 90027

Eastern United States

- ▲ Scientology Missions International
  Eastern United States Office
  349 W. 48th Street
  New York City, New York 10036

United Kingdom

- ▲ Scientology Missions International
  United Kingdom Office
  Saint Hill Manor
  East Grinstead, West Sussex
  England RH19 4JY

Europe

- ▲ Scientology Missions International
  European Office
  Store Kongensgade 55
  1264 Copenhagen K
  Denmark

Africa

- ▲ Scientology Missions International
  African Office
  Security Building, 2nd Floor
  95 Commissioner Street
  Johannesburg 2001
  Republic of South Africa

Australia, New Zealand and Oceania

- ▲ Scientology Missions International
  Australian, New Zealand and Oceanian Office
  201 Castlereagh Street
  Sydney, New South Wales 2000
  Australia

Latin America

- ▲ Scientology Missions International
  Latin American Office
  Federación Mexicana de Dianética
  Pomona 53
  Colonia Roma
  C.P. 06700, Mexico, D.F.

Canada

- ▲ Scientology Missions International
  Canadian Office
  696 Yonge Street
  Toronto, Ontario,
  Canada M4Y 2A7

International Hubbard Ecclesiastical League of Pastors

International Office

6331 Hollywood Boulevard,
Suite 901
Los Angeles, California 90028
Telephone: 213-960-3560
US & Canada: 1-800-HELP-4-YU

Western United States

- ▲ Continental Liaison Office
  Western United States
  1307 N. New Hampshire
  Los Angeles, California 90027

Eastern United States

- ▲ Continental Liaison Office
  Eastern United States
  349 W. 48th Street
  New York City, New York 10036

United Kingdom

- ▲ Continental Liaison Office
  United Kingdom
  Saint Hill Manor
  East Grinstead, West Sussex
  England RH19 4JY

Canada

- ▲ Continental Liaison Office
  Canada
  696 Yonge Street
  Toronto, Ontario
  Canada M4Y 2A7

Africa

- ▲ Continental Liaison Office Afri
  Security Building, 4th Floor
  95 Commissioner Street
  Johannesburg 2001
  Republic of South Africa

Latin America

- ▲ Continental Liaison Office
  Latin America
  Federación Mexicana de Dianética
  Avenida Montevideo 486
  Colonia Linda Vista
  C.P. 07300
  Mexico, D.F.

Australia, New Zealand and Oceania

- ▲ Continental Liaison Office
  ANZO
  201 Castlereagh Street, 3rd Flo
  Sydney, New South Wales 2000
  Australia

Europe

- ▲ Continental Liaison Office
  Europe
  Store Kongensgade 55
  1264 Copenhagen K
  Denmark

Bridge Publications, Inc.
4751 Fountain Ave., Los Angeles, CA 90029
ISBN 0-88404-914-0
NEW ERA Publications International ApS
Store Kongensgade 55, 1264 Copenhagen K, Denmark
ISBN 87-7816-101-0

Printed in the United States of America

An L. RON HUBBARD Publication